EXTREME

Weight Loss Hypnosis
For Women

Learn How to Stop Emotional Eating and Lose
Weight Through Meditation, Hypnosis, Positive
Affirmations and Healthy Eating Habits

By Patricia Lox

TABLE OF CONTENTS

INTRODUCTION

Many women spend their adult lives cycling one after the other through a plan to lose weight, continually ridiculing, and losing weight because of a lack of success. Why do most of us manage every aspect of our life so successfully, but we can't force ourselves to live on a simple diet of loss of weight long enough to increase our health and quality of life?

This is a good question because you should be able to control your weight totally if you can run a business, raise children responsibly and co-ordinate all other aspects of your complicated, fast-paced life!

Hypnosis may help people lose a few pounds, especially diet and exercise when used along with other weight loss methods. Hypnosis is a method of manipulating the state of mind accomplished by controlling a hypnotherapist who uses verbal repetitive mind pictures.

If people are under hypnosis, they are highly concentrated and sensitive to suggestions such as lifestyle changes, which may help to lose weight. Following proper guidance, people may even attempt to hypnotize themselves. Hypnosis of weight loss is also paired with cognitive behavioral therapy. Over the years, several research studies have been carried out to determine their effect on weight loss. Researchers have so far found positive and modest results for weight loss. However, the accuracy of some research was questioned, making it difficult to determine its effectiveness.

Hypnotic condition is like fun relief. Hypnosis is a natural and efficient approach to the subconscious mind, which is the key to unleashing the potential for people, such as changing unwanted habits and behavior and resolving their concerns and problems. Hypnosis is an effective method for inspiring people to lose weight when it comes to weight management. In a study consisting of 60 women who were divided into two groups –

hypnosis and not hypnosis – the group was able to lose an average of 17 pounds. The hypnosis-free group lost only half a pound.

In a separate study, two dietary groups-one used hypnosis, and the other did not-were tracked for two years, which resulted in significant weight loss effects of hypnosis in their diet. There were no significant effects on the other group.

According to others, hypnosis can create beneficial results for a lifetime. A typical session of:

- Induction - The phase to achieve gradual relaxation. This relaxes the muscles from top to top. This allows the conscious mind to relax while the unconscious mind provides the desired suggestions.

- Deepening technique - It sends instructions to the brain to relax more profoundly.

- Imagery - This stage can cause the hypnotherapist to manipulate the mind and body to believe that the visualization is real. Visualization occurs because of certain parts of the brain that can not explain what you see with your eyes and what you see in your mind.

- Suggestions - Once the mind is comfortable, the subconscious mind is flooded with ideas that are very open at this moment.

Eating regularly is just natural, and you will end up eating something that you don't want if you try to restrain yourself. You can learn to eat whenever you want through hypnotism, but you only need to eat healthy food choices and stay away from the fattening foods.

There are also suggestions regarding the multiple possibilities for future research using hypnosis in the field of substance abuse. Suggestions like you only eat to meet the natural need for food as fuel in your body. Repeating these ideas will improve your resolve and increase your sensitivity.

Listening to audio programs with hypnosis, including CDs or tapes, is a well-proven, effective way to treat hypnosis. Hypnosis is a particularly sensitive state of mind. Listen ... Listen ... Those pounds can only be creeping on you, that's for sure. Though it's always the little stuff that adds up.

Ultimately, it becomes automatic, so you may not even know whether or not you locked it without checking. Once this simple habit is in place, it would take an effort to change it. Eventually, this weight loss mindset generated by hypnosis becomes a permanent lifestyle for weight loss. It's best to adopt a "weight loss lifestyle" to lose weight and hold it away; this is what hypnosis promotes.

Studies show that hypnosis is one of the few approaches to weight loss strongly supported by clinical research to promote weight loss successfully. For instance, British researchers have found that there are only two approaches to significant and effective weight loss success in a recent mass analysis of 31 research studies, which cover 13 different common weight loss approaches: hypnotherapy and taking supplements with the illegal substance ephedrine (Pittler & Ernst 2005). Studies show that hypnosis of weight loss and hypnosis of weight control can be very effective. Indeed, some studies have shown that it can be even more effective for men than for women, but only to a limited degree. Studies suggest that people do well on their own rather than by group therapy. To provide more personalized treatment, you may want to see a licensed hypnotherapist.

Work continues to show that women undergo excellent weight training. It develops body strength and, in some cases, helps delay the loss of bones and osteoporosis. Research suggests that in various situations, including after surgery, hypnosis may be helpful for pain and anxiety. Preliminary work suggests that after surgery, hypnotherapy will enhance hospital stay and psychological wellbeing.

Imagine that you can see a short, bent figure walking with

quick, slow steps in the distance. You will most likely conclude that the person is old. Imagine how good it is to get rid of cravings and resolve your unhealthy behavior. Your healthy vision can become a reality by using the most powerful part of your mind (subconscious mind) and my wellness tools. Imagine how satisfied and optimistic you will realize that by years, probably decades, you have prolonged your life and that you have dramatically increased your chances of preventing health issues.

WHAT IS HYPNOSIS?

Hypnosis is the act of leading someone to the state of trance. Various experts describe the trance state differently, but almost always:

- A deep state of relaxation.

- Hyperfocus and concentration.

- Increased suggestibility.

It's because it sounds familiar. Many of us periodically go into and out of the trance state. You are in a trance state when you have zoned out on your normal path, fallen into reverie while listening to music, or find yourself lost in the book or movie universe.

The only difference between hypnosis and this daily trance is that in hypnosis, someone causes the trance to accomplish something: recovery, exploration, or relief from stress, for instance.

What Isn't hypnosis?

What about the part the hypnotist makes you quack like a duck or make your evil bid?

The notion that hypnotists can manipulate their victims' minds and behaviors is a largely media-driven misconception. You monitor all your acts in the trance state; you can hear everything around you, so you can not be compelled to do anything against your will.

Certified Hypnotherapist Cassie Salewske states, "Clients are conscious in a hypnotherapy session, they are awake, they participate, and they recall."

The use of "the power of suggestion" is attributed to hypnosis. However, it is not the only way that our mind is sensitive to suggestion.

"Planting ads, songs, films, and books in our subconscious regularly. Language and communication are full of suggestions, "writes Salewske.

Only participants in stage hypnotism prove that they work in their minds because it is difficult for someone not to be aware of hypnosis.

What Is Hypnotherapy?

Consider hypnosis as a technique and hypnotherapy as the use of a method to explain the difference between hypnosis and hypnotherapy. SAT refers to hypnotherapy as art therapy in practice.

Hypnotherapy is clearly defined by the word itself. Hypnotherapy is the clinical form of hypnosis.

If you are a licensed psychiatrist or psychologist who uses hypnotization to help a patient resolve an emotional or physical disorder, you practice hypnotherapy.

The hypnotic trance is a surprisingly versatile instrument for addressing psychological and physical health problems. Here are just a few examples of using hypnotherapy for mental health and medical professionals:

Helping people avoid smoking or developing alcohol drinking by concentrating their minds and promoting healthy behavior.

Connection to the bond between mind and body to alleviate chronic and acute pain, including surgery and birth. Hypnotherapy has also been shown to be effective against persistent physical disorders such as irritable bowel syndrome and dermatologic disorders.

Immerse yourself in the subconscious mind to identify and treat the root causes of mental health problems like depression, anxiety, PTSD, and addiction. We will concentrate on this last use the rest of this essay. The trance state is the secret to revealing hidden layers in our minds, memories, and intentions, as many hypnotherapists have figured out.

How Does Hypnotherapy Work?

The most important characteristic of the trance state is how our conscious minds are connected to our subconscious minds.
Diane Zimberoff, a co-founder of the Wellness Institute, a pioneer in hypnotherapy, compares the unconscious mind with the computer system. Our subconscious is like our hard drive, which includes all our memories, emotions, and thoughts.
In a calm and hyper-focused state of hypnosis — led by a hypnotherapist — we will go to the root of our mental wellbeing issues by studying Googles into our subconscious.
Zimberoff writes:

- "Any current unhealthy conduct, such as smoking, loss of temper, binge drinking or forced overeating, has a series of events that lays the groundwork for all our current unhealthy choices. The 'memory chip' in our subconscious mind helps us to track the memories and the subconscious choices we have made as children that can lead us to action that is no longer safe for ourselves.

It goes far beyond mere suggestibility. Judi Vitale, an expert hypnotherapist, outlines two very different strategies to help people avoid smoking with hypnotherapy:

- "Using hypnosis, you can help someone quit smoking by saying that the cigarette's taste or smell is worse than it is. However, a hypnotherapist can use age regression to examine the momentum, which fuels the customer's habits and find old results and behaviors. The remedy takes place as the consumer makes new ideas about old memories and prefers new habits rather than smoking.

Vitale says that the second method is much more successful than the first because it is at the root of the problem. Returns come quickly and last.

Does Hypnotherapy Work? What Does the Science Say?

Since it allows direct access to the subconscious mind, hypnotherapy is more effective than conventional recovery approaches for many therapists.

"Hypnotherapy helps us to slip under the logical part of our mind," says Stacie Beam-Bruce, a hypnotherapist. "We can't understand why we do something or why we feel something because it doesn't make sense. Hypnotherapy has access to the emotional convictions of amok.

We recently spoke to 23 qualified hypnotherapists, and everyone said that hypnotherapy had changed their practice and the lives of their clients. In our free ebook, you can read their stories.

But there is more than anecdotal evidence of the workings of hypnotherapy.

"While hypnosis has been controversial, most clinicians now accept that it can be a strong, efficient medical technique for a wide range of conditions, such as pain, anxiety, and mood disorders." The American Psychological Association concludes.

In 2001 a working group was commissioned by the British Psychological Society to review the evidence and to create a comprehensive report on hypnotherapy. 'An array of research now has been accumulated to show that the use of hypnotic approaches may be useful for handling and treating a wide variety of medical, psychological, and psychotherapeutic problems.'

Modern brain imaging technology now provides us with a

panorama of hypnotherapy's physical manifestations. Stanford researchers found that parts of the brain correlated with understanding and improvement showed "changed behavior and connectivity" while analyzing the brains of 57 individuals undergoing hypnosis.

What Mental Health Issues Can Hypnotherapy Help With?

Most of the hypnotherapists trained by the Wellness Institute find that hypnotherapy is most effective in coping with trauma issues.

- "If consumers return to a time when a trauma happened, share their feelings about events and release their emotions, they may time-tamp events that may have plagued them in a way that appears to recreate this traumatic moment," says Vitale.

Hypnotherapist Wendy Pugh tells us that when childhood trauma happened, hypnotherapy works incredibly well.
"My customers have experienced so much healing with hypnotherapy and been able to make so many connections with how their previous traumas affect their current work," she says.
Pugh notes, for instance, that many people do not know how profoundly their present anxieties are embedded in the past.
By analyzing history, feelings are hidden, and the false assumptions found inside the subconscious mind of your clients, you can use hypnotherapy to resolve some of the most vulnerable and persistent barriers to mental health.

How Does Hypnotherapy Work With Other Modalities?

"You are not expected to alter your counseling practice by practicing hypnotherapy radically," says hypnotherapist Catherine Reiss. "The training will encourage you to get to the root of the negative behaviors of your customers and the feelings that they have, but will also help you to use transformation in more conventional formats."

When hypnotherapy has opened the door to the repressed memories and feelings of your clients — months or years of arduous speech therapy formerly — you may use established methods to heal.

"One should start cognitive behavioral therapy and incorporate techniques of trance and hypnotherapy," says Reiss.

Cognitive-behavioral therapy (CBT) supplements hypnotherapy effectively.

How Can You Be Trained in Hypnotherapy?

Hypnotherapy is a strong, scientifically-proven resource to help your customers enter their unconscious minds and solve their most difficult mental health problems. But there are other practical reasons to perform hypnotherapy training as a licensed psychotherapist.

We find, in a recent market survey, that hypnotherapists can easily produce six figures for their practice annually. Hypnotherapy preparation will benefit you, among other financial incentives:

- Charge your services more.

- Reduce references to other providers, and keep more of your patients.

- Insurance panel free break.

- Begin your private practice in a market that is not in use.

How are you going to know hypnotherapy, then? There is no clear route to certification for hypnotherapy, but we suggest to stay away from solo teachers. We typically lack the teaching experience or the network we have with a college or vocational school.
Find an alternative for hypnotherapy training that:
- Is valid for ongoing training loans.

- Certification results (especially relevant for the reimbursement of insurance).

- Is taught by teachers with real expertise in clinical hypnotherapy.

- Incorporates realistic instruction.

HISTORY OF HYPNOSIS

The earliest hypnosis references come from ancient Egypt and Greece. In reality, 'Hypnos' refers to the god and is the Greek word for sleep, while hypnosis is very different from sleep. Both cultures had religious centers where people came to their problems for help. Hypnosis was used to trigger hallucinations, studied to get to the root of the problem. Within early literature, there are also references to trance and hypnosis. In 2600 BC, China 's dad, Wong Tai, has written about techniques involving incantations and handpasses. Hypnotic procedures were described by the Hindu Vedas written around 1500 BC. In many shamanic, druid, audio, yogic and religious practices, trance-like states happen.

Hypnotic Pioneers

Hypnosis' modern father was an Austrian doctor, Franz Mesmer (1734 – 1815), from whose name comes the word 'mesmerism.' Despite being poorly maligned by his day's medical world, Mesmer was nevertheless a brilliant man. He developed the 'animal magnetism' theory – the idea that disease is a result of blockages in the flow of magnetic forces within the body. He felt he might preserve his animal magnetism in iron filings baths and transmit it to patients with rods or 'mesmeric passes.'

The mesmeric pass certainly must go down in history as one of the most interesting and certainly the longest-winded ways to get someone into a trance. Mesmer was standing still for his subjects while he was sweeping his arms over their bodies, sometimes for hours. I suspect that the effect of boring patients into a trance was probably quite effective, but it certainly was. Mesmer himself was a showman, who told the patient in his way that anything should happen. This form of indirect suggestion was quite powerful in itself. Mesmer was also responsible for the hypnotizing image as a man with magnetic eyes, a cap, and a goat's bar. His popularity sparked envy among many of his colleagues, contributing to his public humiliation. Looking back, it is somewhat unbelievable that in the early years' hypnosis had survived since the scientific community was set against it so dead.

John Elliotson (1791–68), a professor at London University, who was famous for bringing the stethoscope to England, was also a progressive thinker. He also tried to defend the use of mesmerism but had to resign. Within his own home, he managed to show mesmerism for all interested parties, contributing to a gradual increase within the literature.

In the mid-19th century, James Braid (1795-1860) was the next true founder of Hypnosis in Great Britain. He developed an interest in mesmerism by chance, primarily a Scottish eye doctor. One day when he was late for an appointment, in the waiting room, he found his patient staring at an old lamp with his eyes sparkling. Fascinated, Braid ordered the patient to close his eyes and go to sleep. The patient was pleased, and the interest in Braid grew. He found that a patient is one of the most critical components to get them into a trance.

The Swinging Watch, which is associated with hypnosis by many people, as common as a fixation in the early days. Braid published a book after his discovery that not all the palaver of mesmeric passes was necessary. He suggested that the process now be referred to as hypnotism.

In the meantime, James Esdaile (1808 – 59), a British surgeon in India, recognized the immense benefits of hypnotic pain relief and conducted hundreds of major operations using hypnotism as the only anesthetic. Once he returned to England, he tried to explain his results to the medical authorities, but they laughed to him and proclaimed pain characteristics (although they preferred modern chemical anesthetics, which they could regulate and charge more money, of course). Hypnosis has since been and remains an "alternative" form of treatment to this day.

The French were also interested in the Hypnosis issue, and numerous breakthroughs were made by men like Ambrose Liébeault (1823 – 1904), J.M. Charcot (1825–93), and Charles Richet (1850–1935), respectively.

The work of Emile Coué (1857-1926), another Frenchman, was quite important. He stepped away from traditional methods and allowed the use of self-suggestion pioneers. He is best known for writing, 'Day by day I get better and better in every way.' His approach was one of encouragement and has been championed in countless modern books.

A man of great kindness, Coué believed that he didn't cure people himself but that he helped to cure himself. He recognized how important it was the involvement of the subject in hypnosis and was a precursor to modern practitioners who say, 'There is no such thing as hypnosis; there is only self-hypnosis.' For example, if you ask someone to pass through a wooden board on the ground, they can do so without wobbling. But if you tell them to close their eyes and think the board is suspended hundreds of feet above ground between two buildings, they start to swing.

In some ways, Coué also predicted the placebo effect – medication of no inherent value that implies that patients are offered a drug that will heal them. Recent placebos research is quite shocking. Statistics sometimes show that placebos can work better than many of the most popular medicines in modern medicine. Although drugs are not always necessary to recover from disease, there seems to be a conviction of recovery.

Sigmund Freud (1856–1939) also took an interest in hypnosis and used it at first. He eventually gave up the practice – not least because he wasn't very good at it for several reasons! He preferred psychoanalysis, which involved a lot of listening by the patient lying on a sofa. He felt the evolution of the self was a complicated process to progress through phases of sexual development with the main cause of psychological disorders being repressed memories of traumatic events. This is an interesting idea that still needs to be demonstrated.

Freud 's early rejection of hypnosis hindered the growth of hypnotherapy, shifting the therapeutic focus away from hypnosis and psychoanalysis. However, in the 1930s, the publication of Clark Hull 's book Hypnosis and Suggestibility shook things up in America.

Previously, Milton H. Erickson, MD (1901-80), a remarkable man and a highly skilled psychotherapist, became the acknowledged leading expert in clinical hypnosis. He was diagnosed with polio and crippled as a teenager, but he pushed himself. He had an exceptional opportunity to observe people when paralyzed, and he noticed that what people said and did was very different. He was fascinated by human psychology and developed several innovative and creative ways of healing people. By metaphor, surprise, uncertainty, laughter, and hypnosis healed. A master of 'indirect hypnosis,' without even using the word hypnosis, he was able to place a person in a trance.

It is increasingly recognized that recognizing hypnosis is necessary for the efficient exercise of all kinds of psychotherapy. Erickson 's approach and its derivatives are the most effective techniques without any doubt.

Over the years, hypnosis in the medical profession has evolved and become respectable. Through hypnosis and medicine are not the same, they are now recognized as related, and it is only a matter of time before hypnosis becomes a common practice acceptable to the public as a dentist 's visit.

GENERAL BENEFITS OF HYPNOSIS

Stop Smoking

When you try to find the perfect way to quit smoking, you'll find the right option with a long list of over-the-counter and prescription nicotine replacement medications and non-nicotine prescriptions. Quitting is, of course, essential: according to the Centers for Disease Control and Prevention, cigarettes are responsible for more than 480,000 deaths a year in the United States. The CDC also estimates that almost seven out of 10 (68 percent) of all U.S. adult cigarette smokers today announced that they want to stop. Herbal treatments, psychiatric medication, and acupuncture are other approaches that are used to stop smoking, but hypnosis was a response to the kick-off of two-packed days for Jon Bryner, a bar owner in Melbourne, Florida (where drinking is still permitted in bars). "They give you a pill when you go to a hospital, but they can't put anti-cloth pills on you," says professional hypnotist Richard Barker. Barker collaborated with Bryner to improve his perspective and to eliminate the emotional attachment to help shift his behavior. "How shall I drive at first, how shall I have a drink and not smoke? "I just think about how horrible smoke feels now," says Bryner.

No More Overeating

Healthier food choices and exercises are the main ingredients for weight loss, but effective weight loss in some situations often requires eliminating emotional and unconscious factors that keep us from losing weight. The use of hypnosis for weight loss involves a different approach to weight loss than for other conditions — it typically takes more than one session to evaluate the specific causes of the patient, explains Barker. "Before hypnosis, I will figure out if they are day-to-day snacks or who hit between meals in the refrigerator. It takes a while for Barker to get out. "Barker sessions continue with embedded commands that help his clients regulate their eating habits. "You close your eyes, after five or six bites, and say 'that's enough' or every time you eat a dish you close your eyes and tell 'eat just half of what's there.'"

Sleep Better

Failure to sleep can impair memory and decision making, which can lead to chronic health issues, including heart disease, obesity, and depression. Although there are several insomnia therapies, including medicine, exercise, and cognitive therapy, it's not easy to think about having enough sleep. Mount Vernon, Washington-based hypnotizer Kelley Woods, states that sleep is controlled primarily by the subconscious. "To try to use conscious thoughts to solve these kinds of problems is like trying to make a corporate change by going to the receptionist — you need to have access to the managing director." "The fear of sleeplessness is what triggers sleeplessness," Barker said. "You'll get a decent night's sleep when you eliminate your fear and worry over not having a good evening." Barker first tells them to imagine a situation where they slept through the night to treat the patients and then use hypnosis to bring them in. "I picture the person getting a good night's sleep in the past, and I make them remove the 'I make insomnia' label and replace it with 'I am sleeping at least eight hours a night.'"

Cure Dental Phobia

The pitchy whirl of the drill, the push of the needle, or simply the discomfort of looking inside the mouth are just some of the reasons people can stop going to a dentist. Although the industry strives to use dental technology to take a ride to the dental clinic less painful, the British Dental Health Foundation estimates that dental anxiety affects about 10 to 20 percent of the world 's population. "Fear has for years driven many of my clients out of the chair," Woods says. "The anxiety may be triggered by a bad dental experience or by listening to someone who has had a negative experience. In any case, it may be compromised, and once it's programmed, the mind may run in default mode. "To help its clients resolve their fear about going to the dentist, it uses neuro-linguistic programming (NLP). "If you start to experience anxiety about going to the dentist, you can use NLP to avoid fear and re-wire your phobia yourself."

Ease Chronic Pain

Pain is a signal which helps us, says Woods, but in chronic pain, even after the body is healed, the nervous system can still relay the pain signal. "We can use hypnotic therapy to dial it down." She recalls a woman with severe back pain who couldn't hold still on the chair. When she asked him what she wanted to do, he said he wanted to put it into wintertime. Woods worked with the client to help him imagine that the bear would rip into a cavern on a snow-caught day, curling up and sleeping. "He describes the pain as a grizzly bear gnawing over his spine. "While hypnosis is not magic, it can sometimes feel like it," Woods says.

Manage Bereavement

If it is a national tragedy or a beloved 's death, a sense of loss or sorrow may weaken, trigger anxiety, insomnia, and depression. Sensing loss by crying helps your mind and body and groups including Mental Health America and the American Psychological Association to help people deal with loss, like thinking about the death of your loved ones, taking care of your health, reaching out to those who experience the loss, acknowledging your emotions and enjoying the life of those that you have. The loss management mechanisms are personal, Barker explains. Hypnotherapy helps to cope with signs of grief by offering constructive thoughts and trying to find ways of coping with loss over time. Barker helps people cope with the loss by putting a "timer" on their sorrow. "Normally, when they are sick and tired of sickness and tired of grief, they let me know."

Relieve Anxiety

Perhaps anyone who deals with anxiety can understand anything because the condition can be worsening and desperate. Anxiety disorders are the most prevalent in psychiatric illnesses affecting more than 25 million Americans, according to the American Psychiatric Association. Although fear is typically treated by medicine or therapy or by a combination of both, many people have become hypnotized. A hypnotist aims to determine whether it's psychological, physical, or based on a past question, the source of stress or anxiety. Barker states that the subconscious mind is what causes you to feel depressed and induces bad habits. "When anyone comes to see me about clogging, clogging is sometimes not a concern; it's anxiety," Barker says. When a man came to Barker for an impediment to speech, he treated him for anxiety.

"His problem wasn't linked to voice, but to his life," Barker said. In the interview, Barker made the man back to the age of six. "He climbed over his house to the roof, and his father screamed at him for being on the roof," Barker says. While the American Stuttering Culture does not accept the claim that stuttering is caused by an emotional phenomenon, Barker thinks it was this incident, the anxiousness of his father shouting combined with the fear of standing on the roof, which led to his impediment to speech. "In the session, I retained the same recollection but changed his father's response from being angry about keeping his arms open and loving him rather than shouting at him. His stammer was gone when he came out of hypnosis.

Stop Tinnitus

Sounds that no one except you can detect is symptoms of tinnitus, a disease 45 million Americans have encountered, according to the American Tinnitus Association, ringing, moaning, or whistling. While tinnitus can be temporary or continuing, most forms of the disorder are not healed. Recovery methods include visual aids, behavior therapy, sound therapy, and TMJ therapy. Hypnosis is an alternative, too. "Tinnitus is caused by the mind," Barker says. "It's because the individual expects it to happen, and the sound goes away until you get rid of the thought of waiting for it."

Make Chemotherapy More Tolerable

One of the earliest known applications of cancer hypnosis occurred in 1829 when M was discovered. Docteur Chapelain used hypnosis to alleviate a breast cancer patient's pain. The doctor used hypnosis as an anesthetic during mastectomy and surgery, while the patient was said to be "calm and showed good pain control." While the standard procedure for surgery is today anesthesia, hypnosis still plays a role in cancer care and is often used to relieve tension and anxiety and alleviate side effects of chemotherapeutics such as nausea and vomiting. "We help you mainly cope with your symptoms and encourage you to improve how you handle pain," said Woods, who deals mostly with cancer patients. "We can not give them false hope, but we can place them safely and encourage them to heal." She says that cancer patients are sometimes moved from doctor to doctor, and they feel like they are a number of them. "We monitor our customers during their chemotherapy appointment, which is a personal encounter with a hypnotherapist that can take a long journey."

Improve Athletic Performance

Michael Jordan, Tiger Woods and Mike Tyson are only some well-known athletes who have turned to hypnosis in their athletic success. Athletes have been using hypnosis long ago to remove negative emotions, de-stress and calm mind and body and improve concentrate and concentration so that they can 'stay in the field.' The therapy will enhance confidence, discipline, and ability and extends to all levels of athletes, including those who rebound from injury and who just learn a sport. "Most athletes go to a hypnotist to improve performance, but they improve their minds," Barker says. "A hypnotist will change your way of thinking and turn your negative habits into positive ones." "To be a good golfer requires a lot of mental stamina," says Barker. "You must alter your perception and reality, and you must both physically and mentally play the game-the the critical mind is locked, but the unconscious mind is in an enhanced condition."

Quicker Recovery From Surgery

Woods uses hypnosis to help patients shorten their recovery period after the procedure, and in some cases, wean themselves off their doctor's prescription pain killers. "I had someone come to me after the procedure, saying that she did not want to live because she was cut off from her opioid supply." Woods used hypnosis in her brain for an explanation of the pain signal. "Thoughts and emotions move in routes, and this is how habits are created," Woods explains. "At first, this is just a road through the woods, but slowly this road becomes a pit you can't get out of." With hypnosis, Woods is forcing the brain and nervous system to follow a different direction. "I needed my patient to live after three sessions."

Ease IBS

The International Federation for Functional Diseases reports that irritable bowel syndrome (IBS) affects 25 to 45 million people in the US. Although the exact cause of IBS is not known, the impact of the disease may vary from mild to weakening. Stress can worsen IBS symptoms, although not the cause of IBS. Although medication varies from probiotics to diets that reduce food triggering – such as low-FODMAP diet – to antidepressants and cognitive behavioral therapy, hypnosis has also been shown to be an effective treatment of IBS in research. Hypnotherapy uses methods of relaxation and hypnotic suggestions to help patients manage their symptoms. The results of the studies showed that the quality of their life and frequent symptoms of abdominal pain, constipation, diarrhea, and bloating have improved.

Immune System Response

Acting with your immune system and controlling it is simpler than you think. You might ask yourself, "Is your immune system influenced? "You 're going to be glad to learn it is.

Most people today understand that the effect of stress on our immune system is negative. They are more likely to become ill and take longer to recover from long-term stress than people who have less stressful lives if they deal with long-term stress. Stress is anticipated in our modern world. Stress management strategies and relaxation protocols can significantly affect your immune system 's health.

The most recent investigation confirms that hypnosis can even boost your immune system. A study at Washington State University gave hypnotic suggestions to a group of volunteers to enhance their immune systems in particular. Another group only received relaxing proposals or no suggestions. A T- and B-cell (special protection cells) levels have been assessed. Those with hypnotic suggestions showed significant increases in their protective cell levels.

Consider this, what makes your heartbeat 100,000 times a day, without you being aware of it? How do the kidneys, liver, and pancreas know what or what to do? How do you know what your stomach and digestive system can do with the food you put in your body?

The autonomous nervous system regulates all the organs, and they operate without telling you what to do and when. Could you imagine how exhausted you would be if you had to spend time each day on all these systems?

Your autonomous nervous system is regulated by your subconscious. In hypnosis, we get direct access to work with you and motivate you to work with the immune system to improve its performance.

Hypnosis is also an effective method for controlling stress and anxiety every day. As you can deal with everyday pressures and problems better, your immune system gets stronger and helps protect weak parts of the body.

When we relax, the brain releases endorphins to restore the balance of the hormone, to control the nervous system, and to encourage a balanced immune system.

Infertility

Yes, hypnotherapy can help you think. Yes, it's real. In the United States, about 6.1 million couples are trying to conceive, and it can take a year or more for many people to get pregnant. It's slightly longer for others.

When we plan to start a family and get pregnant, it's always a burden and worry with our wandering monkey mind that generates all sorts of excuses and causes women to try Google, "Why don't I get pregnant?!" The more irritated, depressed, or worried you get pregnant, the stress hormones your body frees will make you catch a twenty-two so that you do not conceive as early.

It's like your body wants you to be calm and able to embrace the responsibility that you ask for before it takes place. Hypnotherapy may be an ideal alternative or complementary treatment to allow you to feel confident with your first child. Hypnosis will help you to feel more confident, relaxed, and better handle stress every day.

This prevents the body from releasing adrenaline and cortisol hormones into the bloodstream. So much of these hormones can make it difficult to conceive as they interfere with the brain portion that regulates other hormones. The only one who will profit from hypnotherapy is not Mom-to-be.

The stress of infertility will reduce Dad's level of testosterone and the consistency of semen, making the whole thing much more complicated for you both. Hypnotherapy can lead to fertility issues by helping both mother and dad to feel calmer, more relaxed, and controlled, and thereby reduce stress and anxiety.

Seasonal and Food Allergies

Hypnosis is a highly effective (no side effects) remedy in the fight against environmental and food allergies. Allergies in springtime, such as hay fever, are caused by an acute reaction or allergic pollen reaction. Hay fever (like any allergy) is an immune system overreaction. The immune system wrongly identifies the pollen as a threat and produces an unwanted reaction.

Techniques in clinical hypnosis will benefit you in three main ways:

- Allergy-related pain relief and allergic reactions.

- Educating an immune system about friendly and unfriendly environmental chemicals or substances and restore the sense of biochemical safety with the subconscious mind.

- Avoid overreacting to toxins and allergic reactions to other foods in the body.

WEIGHT LOSS HYPNOSIS AND WOMAN

Hypnosis can best be known as the party trick used to make people dance chicken on stage, but more and more people turn to the technique of mental stimulation to help them make better decisions and lose weight. Case in point: When Georgia, age 28, chose in 2009 to lose 30 or so pounds, the dietary veteran went back to hypnosis. The mental management strategy had led to her overcoming a fear of flying and hoped it would also help her to make good eating habits.

At first, the self-proclaimed food was shocked by the advice of her hypnotherapist. "[She had] four simple rules that I would have to accept: eat when you're hungry, listen to your body, eat what you want, stop when you're full, slowly eat and have a full mouth," explains Georgia. "As such, I was not allowed to eat anything in mild music to my ears!"

Who Should Try Hypnosis

Hypnosis is a gentle way for someone to lose weight and become a habit. Isn't it for one person? Anyone interested in a quick fix. Reframing unhealthy food thinking takes time-her hypnotherapist tells Georgia eight times a year, and it took a month to begin seeing a real improvement. "The weight fell slowly and gradually, without any drastic adjustments in my lifestyle. I still eat several times a week, but mostly sent food back on me. I enjoyed my food for the first time and had time to drink tastes and textures. Almost oddly enough, I had re-entered my love affairs with food so that I could lose weight," she says.

How to Use Hypnosis to Lose Weight

Hypnosis is not meant as a "diet," but instead as a method to help you excel in consuming and exercising healthy food, says Traci Stone, Ph.D., MPH, ASCH-certified clinical psychologist in Columbia University and former Director of Integrative Medicine in the Columbia Department of Surgery. Hypnosis helps people experience how they feel when they are strong, fit and in control, and overcome their mental barriers to achieve these objectives in a multi-sensory manner, "she says. Hypnosis can help people solve the psychological problems underpinning them so that they can hate exercises, experience intense cravings, binge at night, or eat carelessly.

Hypnosis is helpful not to be considered a diet, says Joshua E. Syna, MA, and LCDC, a certified hypnotherapist at the Houston Hypnosis Centre. "This works because it transforms the way they think about food and food, and it allows them to learn to be calmer and happier in their lives. Thus, rather than eating and food becoming an emotional response, it is an effective solution to hunger, and new behavior habits have been created that make it easier for the individual to cope with emotions and life." "Hypnosis works to reduce weight because it allows a person to separate food from emotional life."

Dr. Stein says the use of self-guided audio programs produced by a qualified hypnotist (look for the ASCH certification) is fine for people without any other mental health problems. But beware of all the new applications on the online market-one study has found that most applications are untested and often make grandiose claims about their effectiveness that can not be proved.

What Hypnosis Feels Like

Forget about what you saw in films, and on stage, therapeutic hypnosis is closer to treatment than a circus trick. "Hypnosis is a joint experience and every step of the way the patient should be well informed and comfortable," says Dr. Stein. And she adds that for people concerned about being fooled into doing something odd or dangerous, you should not even do something under Hypnose. "It's only concentrated attention," she explains. "Each person goes into light trance states several times a day naturally – think of when you are out, as a friend shares every detail of her holiday – and hypnosis simply learns to focus this inner attention effectively."

Dispelling the myth that hypnosis seems strange or frightening from the patient's side, Georgia always says she felt very clear and controlled. There were also funny moments like when we were told to watch her weight move on the scale. "My extremely imaginative imagination had to imagine removing all of the clothing, all the rings, my watch, and my hair clip until I was jumping on in the nude. Everyone else does that, or is it just me?"

The One Downside of Hypnosis for Weight Loss

It is not intrusive; it fits well with other therapies for weight loss and does not require any tablets, powders, or other supplements. Something happens at the worst, putting it in the camp "could help, can't hurt." Yet Dr. Stein acknowledges that there is one downside: quality. Costs per hour vary but range from $100 to $250 an hour for clinical hypnosis services, and when you see the therapist once or more per week for a month or two, it can add up quickly. And most insurance undertakings do not support hypnosis. However, Dr. Stein says it can be compensated if it is included in a broader mental health care program, so consult with your provider.

A Surprising Perk of Weight Loss Hypnosis

Hypnosis is not only emotional, but it's also a medical aspect, says Peter LePort, MD of the MemorialCare Center for Obesity in California. "You must first deal with any underlying weight gain metabolism or physiology, but by using hypnosis, you may develop healthy behaviors," he says. And hypnosis is another positive thing: "The therapy element can also help relieve tension and increase concentration, which can help to lose weight in turn," he says.

So Does Hypnosis Work for Weight Loss?

There is an astounding number of scientific research that explores the effectiveness of hypnosis in terms of weight loss. The initial research, published in 1986, found that women who used a system of hypnosis lost 17 pounds compared to 0.5 pounds for females who were advised to look at what they eat. In the 1990s, the meta-analysis of weight loss studies showed that subjects who used hypnosis lost about twice the weight. And in a 2014 study, women who used hypnosis enhanced weight, BMI, eating habits, and even other aspects of their body's image.

But it's not all good news: A Stanford study in 2012 showed that around a quarter of people simply couldn't be hypnotized and it has nothing to do with their personalities, contrary to popular belief. Instead, the brains of certain people don't seem to work that way. "If you're not prone to daydreaming, often find it difficult to get stuck in a book or take a seat in the movies, and don't feel creative, then you may become one of those who don't work well with hypnosis," says Dr. Stein.

Georgia is a success story. He claims it motivated her not only to lose extra pounds but also to hold her safe. Six years on, she happily maintained her weight loss, even going in when she needs a refresher with her hypnotherapist.

HYPNOSIS CLEARS THE METABOLIC PROGRAMMING THAT PREVENTS WEIGHT LOSS

If you are overweight, you may be sick of reminding people that losing weight means consuming less food and getting fewer calories. You may have tried both old and new diets. Yet it also seems that our bodies have found a way to turn a lettuce plate into a pound of fat! Many people who want to lose their weight sooner or later find out that aerobic systems that keep their weight on the body regardless of whether their eating patterns change hinder their efforts.

If you or your friend or client is overweight, and you want to see how these services impact weight loss efforts, take the following questionnaire:

- Should you eat less than your slim mates and don't lose weight?

- Are you looking for food cravings just when the pounds continue to fall off? As if you were hungry rather than dietary?

- Are you exhausted and lethargic while you diet?

- Do you find that the weight doesn't just fall as fast as it should, no matter how much you starve?

- Are you gaining all your weight back from an alarming-speed diet?

If you replied "yes" to one of these questions, you probably have a subconscious metabolism to retain your body weight instead of consuming it for energy.

Here are the good ones now! There are several ways we can approach this system by hypnosis to stop battling the body and food cravings to lose weight!

First, the possible causes of this programming must be investigated.

The metabolism of food is the dynamic mechanism by which the body absorbs and uses nutrients from food. This is a dynamic mechanism involving a variety of variables. One is the thyroid gland feature, the 'master' switch that controls the cell metabolism levels. Via hypnotic imaging, the main metabolic hormone released by the thyroid gland, thyroxine, is released. More thyroxine means more fat has been consumed, and more energy has been lost to you. There may be medical causes for thyroid dysfunction, but before going into hypnotherapy, we recommend a full physical evaluation and a potential check for thyroid function.

The development of two main pancreatic hormones, insulin and glucagons, is another essential factor in body metabolism processes. Such primary metabolic hormones hold or burn our body fat. The foods you consume affect the activities of these hormones directly. In general, most carbohydrates, including sugars, tend to cause insulin secretion, which increases the metabolism of sugar and storage. Glucagons, which are secreted after a low-carbon meal, allow the body to consume protein and d fat, including fat stores of the body. This is part of why low carb diets are popular.

So how does hypnosis help you change your eating choices?

Since all eating habits are ingrained in the unconscious, consciously choosing to eat differently is rarely enough to make changes in our food habits in the long term. The image of hypnosis targets and adjusts these subconscious programs in a way that is both stable and almost straightforward. Personal hypnotic scripts that can be written on a self-hypnosis tape and heard in bed every night can be produced by working with a hypnotherapist.

Exercise is also an essential component of metabolism activation. Studies have discovered that daily exercise not only speeds up metabolism during the workout but even for hours, even when you rest, often for as little as 30 minutes a day. Of course, many of us have trouble exercising. Join the power of hypnosis again. Hypnotic ideas can be used to improve motivation and strength and stamina for physical activity. Most sometimes, it takes, even more, to get interested in exercise than simple hypnotic advice.

Some of the creative methods we use will lead you back to what you like to do as a child. You can choose one or two of the activities you will enjoy again! We use the power of hypnosis to bring back your excitement as a child. We can also go back to these painful encounters, which have made us turn to the joys of physical activity to save the past from these traumas. For example, an experience of being rejected, humiliated, or hurt on the playground in a team sport may cause one to avoid playing outside. Our rescue mission enables the child to receive comfort and promise of self-assurance from an adult and an invitation to play with the adult on the outside.

Genetic is one of the most common sources of metabolic programming. Some human genetics (South Pacific Islanders and Eskimos are only two extreme examples) retain fat more readily on their bodies, for thousands of years in particular during famines, these traits have served their forefathers well. This can be difficult for even qualified clinicians to alter certain genetic codes in our DNA. We may, however, convince the metabolism to bypass these DNA programs through hypnosis and help us get fat. Once my clients told me, "My whole family is overweight." Now is the time to use such hypnotic techniques to bypass DNA programming.

Another common concern with those dealing with weight loss is that the subconscious mind can fear weight loss, and if weighing concerns are absent, even scarier issues will potentially be experienced. One client told me in trance that she would have to "do something about my life, and I don't know what I would do!" If she was losing this weight, she was fascinated with it. At the Institute, we could check these issues and provide a therapeutic plan. One useful strategy to use here is a trip to the future individual to explore how one's life goal can be accomplished.

Another common issue I discovered among women who use metabolic programming to stay fat is that their bodies need to isolate themselves from fat to protect themselves from undesired sexual progress. Most of my obese clients are victims of sexual exploitation during childhood. And others have gained weight to hide their unsatisfied sexual desires. Others use weight as an excuse for not meeting people and thus face dismissal or treason. It could be in the subconscious mind deeply buried and still affect your metabolism if you are not aware of such unconscious programming. Your hypnotherapist will help you discover these issues and cure them. I have personally been very active in saving clients from early sexual assault, which also resulted in a dramatic loss of weight without any noticeable change in diet.

5 KEY REASONS WOMEN GAIN WEIGHT AND THE TECHNIQUES YOU CAN USE TO OVERCOME THEM

When it comes to food, as with almost anything these days, options are abundant. Especially if you live in a big city, the number of restaurants, cafes, fast food joints, popcorn stands, grocery stores, and markets have never been this huge. It requires immense willpower not to give in to temptation and indulge whenever hunger hits – or simply when something looks or smells delicious. But the thing is, availability is just part of the problem. The problem when it comes to overeating, or eating badly, goes even deeper.

Besides, five main areas need to be discussed when it comes to effectively using hypnosis for weight loss. In this chapter, we 're going to take an in-depth look at these issues and the hypnosis methods you can use to solve each of them.

However, to get the most out of this chapter, we suggest that you don't cheat and take the time to read it in full!

So put the kettle on, pull up a chair, and get ready to discover how you can successfully use hypnosis for weight loss.

1. The Relationship Your Subjects Have With Food & Their Food Culture

Every culture has a link to food. Food is important for all living beings, but it is especially important for humans. This has social implications, and routines are around it. It is a crucial point in life. Whoever you are, where you live, or in what kind of setting you have been born, food has played a part in your everyday life. If you think about it, it makes sense. After all, food is part of a ritual for most people in the developed world three times a day: breakfast, lunch, and dinner. Many people underestimate the value of food in their lives by saying things like: "I'm just living to live on. I just want to take a pill to live on."

But this feeling is more the exception than the law. To most people, food has a wide variety of definitions and connections – some of them when you could barely walk. Take a little girl at the table with her food, for instance. What's her mom saying?

"It's a good girl to eat all your dinner."

"Hey, mommy, I don't want to."

"Tell mom how much you love her by plate clearing."

What was not there? Who wasn't? It's hard to be a mom. Especially when you have a child when they begin to break boundaries, it is enough to test everyone's patience, and you will use any tactics you need to ensure your child gets all the nutrients it needs even if you have to make use of remorse.

It isn't the world's end, right? Okay, you see, the problem is that it produces a bond in mind. Food is like passion. Nutrition is how I give love or how I give myself to be loved. If a child grows up, he or she may lead the idea to his or her own adult life. They get married, and how do they show the extent of their love for their partner? By spoiling them as much as they can with food.

The reasoning behind it can be a bit like this:

Did it have a bad day? For your favorite cake, let me surprise you!

And while your intentions are fine, your waistlines and your wife – not to mention long-term health – paint another picture. Food is at the center of festivities in most cultures. Birthdays, marriages, bar mitzvahs, birthdays, holidays, anniversaries and the list continues. Nearly every special opportunity revolves around food.

You get a promotion, for example. You may join your chosen university. You land the dream job for which you have applied. How do you do? How do you do? You go out to share a meal and a bubble bottle. Food has a different significance depending on its history. For example, food plays an enormous ritualistic and social role in some African cultures. To understand the relationship of a topic to food, you need to understand the society in which they have evolved or in which they now belong.

One way to find out more is to ask questions. Here are some examples of the kind of questions you can ask which reveal the cultural food references and preferences of a subject:

"What did your parents tell you when you were young?" (The usual strong responses here are guilt, shame, and love).

"Why did you celebrate with food? Did you enjoy food and eat together?" (Food is also related to happy occasions or significant milestones).

"Is food a crutch when bad things happen?" (this illustrates how their feelings affect the food relationship.)

You can have to dig deep to figure out how the culture of a country affected the way they think about food.

How To Overcome Issues With Food Culture

It isn't a problem for someone who doesn't have a specific food culture to grow up. Food is just fuel for them. You 're eating it, or you're not consuming it. Nonetheless, things are different for others. They may have grown up with food connected with love, shame, or guilt in a family. The perfect example is when parents in the first world say their kids don't waste their food. "African children are hungry." Again you have to ask questions about your hypnosis subjects. Specifically, around: "What kind of things your parents said when you grew up about food? Several instances are as follows:

- Have they ever used the line of 'starving children in Africa?'

- Have you ever been told to consume more, and if they did, how can they consume more?

- Have you ever been celebrating with food?

- Have you ever devoted yourself to food?

- Why did you and your parents use food that grows up?

- What do you mean?

- What is healthy food for you?

There are several issues, as you can see. This is a longer conversation that can take up to one hour depending on the form of relationship with food that people developed as part of their community. The goal is to remove the reference points to find out where they come from. If this is possible, the next step is a reframing.

There are a variety of ways to reframe, but it is best to start with the easiest, the least invasive, and only climb up if you are rejected along the way. An example of an incredibly simplistic journey is the starving children in Africa, the shame trip. You may answer this with a de-frame test, which challenges the fundamental logic of the idea.

For example, to suggest that you should eat because children in Africa are starving and you waste food is a major guilt trip.

The question to ask, however, is: is that true?

Why would it help a hungry child in Africa if you finish anything on your plate? Alternatively, how does it affect a starving child in Africa if you waste any food on your plate? You can see that this basic de-frame is already eroding the definition. The next thing to do is to look at what is happening. Once you finish everything on your plate and particularly once it is an over-dimensional plate, what you're going to do is spread out your butt. Your stomach is supposed to be a dimension roughly the size of a palm. Nevertheless, other stomachs are the size of many palms, and the more you feed, the more they grow. Then it takes more calories to fill the stomach as it is larger.

Within this deframe, you will bring up some embedded suggestions to inject the idea into your unconsciousness. You might say something like this, for example:

The act of finishing what is on your plate, even though you are already happy, even if you feel full already, is your only human. You will have extra food in your body that creates fat that affects your wellbeing, and that will enlarge your stomach in the long term. Over the long term, you should be more hungry and continue to consume more food. You pick up the part of "feel hungry," implying it will take longer before you feel fulfilled.

You add the concept of feeling fulfilled and end up eating more food that they do not need. Where is the food going? On their paws, it could lead to medical problems. It's not just wrong that they hurt kids by not consuming it all; they hurt themselves.

They can also benefit the environment because the more food they consume, the less excess food in impoverished areas. It is the rationale to question and defraud the premise. There are other ways to support poor children in Africa, other means of celebration, and other forms of fellowship. There are other ways the feelings can be handled. This emphasis on their culinary culture is something that can be demonstrated as a discussion leads to it and not something that you need solely to spend a session on.

Also, if they get stuck on the thought, during the deframe task, then you might try to open up something like Mind Bending Language and return to the frame so that they can reshape their relationship with food again. If that doesn't work for whatever cause, regression will be the next move.

The re-imprint, which is a hypnotic re-education process, is a fantastic regression model in these cases. When their minds realize that finishing everything on their plates is terrible for them and the world, they have to go back and symbolically inoculate their younger version with a re-print to help them restore themselves.

The re-imprint method is a kind of regression plus. The aim is to incorporate skills into it, which can be depended upon in the future, such as the opportunity to say no to food if it is excessive. The trick here is to repeat this pattern over time so that the pattern is absorbed into your mind. And just to be sure, when we say in time, we mean that during the regression, you should give the child the suggestion. And you should repeat this suggestion as you unconsciously grow up your inner boy. You are going to drive them through late childhood, adolescence, young adulthood right up to the moment repeating the suggestion. You should show them how to think about these issues in this way.

Note: We recommend a 3-6 month regimen if we use hypnosis for weight loss. Often it takes even a year to fix food issues when they occur. Through this time, your subject will undergo birthdays, festivals, and ultimately even loss or death. You can also be blamed or shamed by family and friends. The root cause of the issue takes time and discusses attitudes and habits, and it is better to deal with them organically. Yet if you help them cope with these issues, they will lead a safer and happier life.

2. The Relationship Your Subject Has With Food and Their Emotions

This is a big category that can theoretically be dealt with in one session – or multiple sessions that take to be completely identified. The goal is simply to explore the relationship of your subject with your emotions and exaggeration. This is, of course, a rather profound question at one point. Yet before you can lose weight, you don't have to be a Buddha, who contemplates life on a rock. The question is that people are using food to combat negative emotions.

If you have a lot of tension in your life, you find comfort in sugar. It is because stress is consumed by sugar (in the form of glucose reserves) like nothing else, and it needs to be substituted. Such stores of glucose are the emergency supplies of the body. As soon as you kill them, the body enters the super hungry state to replace them. If people are too stressed out, glucose burns very quickly. This always makes them hungry, and they eat at the candy bars constantly and the like to replace the food they have lost.

Plus, there is another issue when you feel depressed or weak. You see, you want your body to regulate your mood by releasing serotonin, otherwise referred to as the "good hormone."

All right, should you be thinking? While its motives are good, it can contribute to a strong appetite for sugar – which is the way your body develops serotonin. Therefore, it is important to consume certain foods that produce naturally serotonin as well as protein and fermented food and drink, such as B6 products (e.g., spinach, salmon, celery, tuna, and poultry). Yet there is also another problem with the stress that goes beyond what someone puts into their bodies.

You can see that you release three hormones when you are stressed: cortisol, adrenaline, and norepinephrine. These hormones are also responsible for your fight or flight response when you are worried about a potential threat. And because of the perceived danger, your body sticks to fat if, for example, you need it in an emergency if you run out of food. While this was a convenient way for our great ancestors, it is less necessary today if a saber-toothed tiger eventually cornered them into a cave for days. Normally, it causes extreme stomach blowing, and studies have also shown that it is difficult to lose weight with long-term stress. It's a vicious cycle that is intensified because the body is more used to consuming glucose than fat. Ironically, fat is the higher (and longer-lasting) fuel.

There are other emotional elements to consume, aside from pain. People use food to set down negative feelings. Take, for example, the standard North American stereotype of the man or woman dumped. The man who gets dumped goes out to comfort himself with his friends and alcohol and forgets his troubles. He eats pizza and drinks beer the majority of the day. The woman who is dumped can go out on white wine with the ladies, or stay home and binge on chocolate and ice cream.

Such assumptions have become deeply entrenched, in part because of the influence of ads. Anyone who uses these principles will certainly sell his goods to us.

"You lead a life of quiet despair? Everything didn't work out as you would have hoped? Never mind. Never mind. Buy this 6-pack beer or huge tub of ice cream, and it will look a lot better.

Note: In addition to alcohol, which is typically not a successful solution to cope with the difficulties of life, do you know that it contains seven calories a gram? Where are four calories per gram of carbohydrates and protein and nine calories per gram of this fat? Anything to focus on during the next snap, you open a 6-pack.

Depression is another emotion that can contribute to weight gain. Biochemical and psychological causes are very closely related to depression and weight gain. You must be cautious when coping with depression, as your country's laws can forbid it as part of your treatment. And even though someone thinks – rather than becoming clinically stressed – this may also lead to poor food decisions and a downward spiral. What you want is consistency in every plan that deals with weight loss and weight management to guarantee that you face the emotional side of things. You set yourself and your subject to excel in this way.

For example, gastric band hypnosis is currently becoming very interesting. This is based on the conceptual concept of a physical gastric band, a medical operation that puts an elastic band around the belly to reduce its thickness. They end up with a tummy that is half as big so that they get stronger and eat less potentially.

But the gastric band surgery is an issue. It is a physical restraint in the stomach. If you eat a little too much, you can still expand the part of the stomach that has not been removed. It will grow and expand over time until it is right back from where it began. If you don't care about the emotional elements, a person can do almost anything.

The unconscious mind can ignore reality, whether it's healthy or unhealthy for a larger purpose. The same applies to the hypnotic version. If you don't care about the emotional component, you can risk sabotaging everything else, because you create conflict.

The management of the emotional component is the most critical of the five reasons discussed in this chapter. If you are right, all else tends to come into play nine times out of 10. You will hopefully try to help them develop a whole new way of life around food and their food choices.

How To Overcome Emotional Issues With Food

Again, you can continue stuff with questions. For example: For example:

- How happy are you about your life?

- How happy are you with 1-10 scales? With ten beings, "I feel so grateful that I wake up with joy in the morning," that one being, "I wake up in the morning and wonder why I'm living only because I don't see it."

Note how difficult the questions are since most people are going to be right in the center. Most citizens are not unhappy, but neither are they extremely pleased. Now you have to figure out what is missing.

Note: If a subject is particularly depressed, it could be (and necessary) best to refer it to a medical practitioner who deals with depression first.

If they are five, what are the missing 5 points that will make them 10? Usually, two items are to be searched for, either what is missing or what is present that keeps them from going on. Stressors may be the product of a challenging job or manager, problems about relationships, financial difficulties, or difficulties with a child.

What is lacking can be linked to life decisions. You may feel like you have opted for something you did not want, or you're stuck in a career choice and fear moving. Both these stimuli can lead to irritation and maybe even more tension. At a certain angle, these aspects can be changed simply by making more of their lives.

However, as a hypnotist, the job is to encourage people to lead better lives and not to inspire them.

To do so, you must focus on two things:

- How to treat issues, come back and rebound from stress – and do so in a positive way.

- How to lead a healthier lifestyle, live a happier everyday life.

There are a few methods that you can use to accomplish these two. The challenges of deframing and reframing can play a significant role in the production of emotions. That is because people sometimes misinterpret their lives in such a way as to stress them. Essentially, they assign greater significance to the actions of other people and turn their lives into a soap opera. Soap operas are nuts. Soap opera. A land of violent chaos and relentless drama. But it is cheap drama, a highly emotional drama, written to keep you occupied. If someone's rude to you – and from a soap opera point of view you see things – you can find them a jerk. It's more than one dimension: they've done something for me.

Nonetheless, this person could only have a bad day in real life. He or she may have lost focus because they have had bad news. You should go to the hospital for an emergency. Two subjective assumptions are very distinct. The guy is a jerk, on the one hand. They 're having a bad day, on the other hand. You must know how they came to an emotional conclusion by questioning it.

The NLP Meta Model is really strong. You will learn a lot more by asking questions like:

- What happened makes you believe it's happening?

- What makes you think they think about you?

- How are you aware?

- What makes you believe it's a real direct assault on you?

It may or may not be an actual attack. When it's unclear, it is easier not to note an attack than to deal with it. Why? Why?
And if it's passive, it isn't detrimental to ignore. The only one who gets hurt is the passive aggressor because they are ignored, and if they are, what will the answer be?
It will be some sort of wrath, rage, or fear as they become tangled. Most of the time, people build their drama in a certain way by looking at the universe. Regression is a key component here, particularly when they are more anxious, nervous, and depressed due to trauma in the past. There is a direct connection between severe and unexplained trauma. This trauma can be like sexual assault, abandonment, or neglect. This could be an accident or a tough time. When they are weak in their teens and don't always have enough to eat, they vow never to starve again when they are older and richer.
Those kinds of promises can be partly cultural and partly emotional, and they combine. To deal with this, a regression or re-imprint can be useful. You might, for example, re-print a pseudo-childhood that was full of abundance. This will do much to restore their present moment, when abundance is their reality, even though they may not feel it.
Rebirth is what it takes for most people. They will look from a different angle at their everyday problems. What happened this week? What happened? It happened, it occurred, and it occurred. So you are reviving moments of achievement, moments of pride, moments of good results, and ability to interact with people. Let's assume; for example, someone has been broken by their boss. They broke into tears and went home and had an ice cream drink.

So you're reviving stuff they were doing, like helping a worker on the street, working in a charity, and doing something positive for someone else and feeling good about it. If you revive them, take them to the degree that they are very pleased with how strong they are. Then give them an image to reflect the revival, for example:

- Which kind of person does that?

- Which kind of person does that help?

- What kind of person supports co-workers, kitchen volunteers, is smart socially, etc.?

You might assume he's a loving person, a compassionate person, or an intelligent person. Very. Very. They are beneficial stickers. They are the equivalent of a conversational signal. And you might wonder how a kind and an intelligent person might have responded to the wrath of your boss? All you are doing is releasing tools to revive the issue in the last few minutes. The question is the frustration and the desire to cope. They 're motivated right now. So this is the PCAT formula in practice but in a more conversational way.

If you don't feel comfortable talking and doing it honestly, you can use classic hypnotic activators to restore positive self-success and power experiences in general. It's a more straightforward and equally successful approach:

"Okay. Go back to your boss. He's screaming at you. Feel this. See what is going on now."

You can also chat freely about a positive occurrence that has little to do with the problem you are faced with inside a coaching system. The challenge lies in the optimistic environment of this experience.

For example:

"I wonder what your situation will tell you about this experience?"

They might tell at first: "Nothing."

If so, question them more by saying: "Think about it."

You need to be certain because you can see something they don't see: "Think hard about it. I think you lack something."
So they begin to wonder:
"Oh, perhaps."
"Move ahead." "Go on."
"Oh, maybe that."
"Improve it a little more."
We will link themselves, bit by bit. Suddenly, they say: "Oh my Gosh. It's like ..." As you get there, you realize that you're hitting "T" in the PCAT formula, and the transition stage is full. We will initially be sluggish and tentative, so wait. You know it begins to take until they make links, and their excitement explodes.
And note the feeling will always be a significant part of what you do. This is the backbone of every plan for weight loss. Get this part right, and everything else will be enforced.

3. Your Subject's Understanding Of Nutrition & Their Genetics

It wasn't a concern in the past, but with the range of foods now available, it is becoming increasingly so. This is because food can be confusing. To most people, following the dietary recommendations to food packaging is not so straightforward.
Furthermore, fast food ensures that children don't need to cook for themselves. We go to more restaurants and engage in the fast-food culture. You eat pre-cooked food. They are not chefs; they are reheaters. Stick to the microwave, stick to the oven, stick to a pot, or position on the burner. Even if they don't, they 're going out for a meal or brought away.
What are these things problems? Okay, first of all, a lot of food is not healthy for you at the restaurant. They put stuff into it that makes it enticing, so you return, but health is not always their priority. The flavor that makes you spend more money on

the next cheesecake.

Secondly, the same applies to the food industry packed. Your company is to sell canned food, and you can put it on garbage if you want to buy it. Most of it is sugar like an open invitation to diabetes and related diseases, in the form of high-fructose maize syrup.

We add sugar to our biology because it's uncommon in the wild. This is a valuable source of energy that is also very addictive. Research indicates that sugar activates the same portion of the brain as alcohol, cocaine, and tobacco. So don't make a mistake: it can be very addictive. And if a food producer can make you dependent on their commodity, you will buy more.

The result is that they don't know how or though people try to eat healthily. The belief that fats make you fat, for example, is probably not true. Yeah, consuming more fat than burning can contribute to weight gain. Nevertheless, healthy fats are better for the development of the brain and are, of course, superior to refined fats. Many have tried and ended up being worse to take all the fat out of their diets for the sake of a diet.

Why? Why? Since healthy fat is an essential nutrient that indirectly converts into your fat. It must be torn down and restored– not just from one to the next. As a hypnotist who deals with weight loss issues, it is critical that you give nutritional advice to your subjects. Otherwise, they won't be able to make healthy food decisions that help them build the kind of lifestyle that regulates their weight.

One of the big things to remember is the importance of ethnic heritage. Northern Europe, for example, is a very cold climate, not suitable for plants and fruits. It's perfect for meat and heavy dairy diet, and the genetic making of the people who live there is strong lactose production.

Southern Europe has a very mild and cool climate in countries like Spain and Italy. There is plenty of fruit and vegetables that are easy to produce. People in this part of the world tend to have a digestive system that is perfect for fructose and so on. Yet they are more vulnerable to lactose intolerance and related issues. Therefore, nutrition is not a single-size equation. The genetic history of your subject has a role to play. Take the Inuit, for instance. Their diet consists of 50% fat, mostly whale and seal blubber. Yet their bodies should live with it. They need to stay dry!

There are hypnotic methods that you can use to help them lose weight, but also some basic nutritional science. The enzymes in the body have been engineered for thousands of years to manage the foods that their ancestors might find locally. People learned to specialize and consume the sort of food they needed to supply all the nutrients.

And it may also vary from person to person from Northern Europe to Southern Europe.

This is why a mixture of foods that may work for another person might not work for you. Perhaps it is not the best mix for your heritage.

It's a hard thing to absorb. This doesn't only happen in the heart, but primarily in your chest. The cycle includes a lot of bacteria, including probiotics, including enzymes. There is a different flora for every human.

The more you harm your intestines, the more damage there is, and the more you will have to endure a scheme to repair some part before you turn to another part. And if you experience a major physical transition, like pregnancy, you will note changes too. What are some typical things that are associated with pregnancy, particularly with food choices, apart from morning sickness?

You've got special cravings. But why? But why? Since they feed two, and the baby requires other nutrients. A baby consumes multiple resources such that the mother's nutrients and vitamins are reduced by two of them. The problem is not the amount; it is the mineral content or nutritional content. The body is a perfect laboratory to detect the quality of food. That is why we like chocolate and potato chips because the body is like sugar and salt. It's very difficult to get into the wild, and sugar is a cheap and quick source of energy if you get it. That's one of the reasons why people gorge on it.

Through pregnancy, a woman's body detects the loss of certain minerals and is keen to recover them. If you want such odd things, like the rubber scent on concrete, it is because certain aromas or aromas have caused the body to anticipate those nutrients. It is where the drive comes from.

And there is an easy way to test this when it comes to food intolerances. It's the rate of pulse. If you eat something of which you are intolerant, your heart speeds up. Your pulse increases as the body get irritated by being poisoned quite slightly.

How To Enhance A Subject's Understanding Of Nutrition

Food is our first real component of actions. In other words, you want to change your subject's way of making food. It is necessary to have some training so that you can better advise them. There is, of course, plenty of material online, but don't get pulled into current fads.

Only put your food groups, proteins, carbohydrates, fats, minerals and vitamins, and understand. People need balance. Proteins, including carbohydrates, proteins, fats, vitamins, and minerals, do many things. You have to speak to your subjects about this to make sure they know what these things are, what they do with them, and what food is healthy.

When you talk about nutrition, for example – most people talk about beef. Beef has a pretty high protein content, but non-meat protein sources are not taken into account by most people. These include nuts, eggs, and Parmesan cheese, that has crazy protein, and believe it or not.

What you do is provide options for people, make them interested, and encourage them to create new food choices. When you can get them curious about food, they can teach themselves a lot about food. The aim is to be sarcastic, to taunt them with an insane food reality, and then annoy them to prove their error. To get them to look up and then realize it's true:

"Look. It's on Wikipedia. It's on this MD site. It's on this food site. It's real." It must be real.

They are starting to be excited by the truth about food and nutrition. They provide nutrition in their conversation. They put nutrition on their reticular triggering device, the part of the mind that takes care of things. This is a priority. What you don't want is to avoid eating wrong, something called orthorexia. You want them to recognize food classes so that they enjoy a healthy diet.

You may not survive without carbohydrates, for example, but slow carbs and fast carbs exist. Slow carbs such as beans and potatoes last for longer and give you sustained energy while fast carbs such as candy and popcorn only provide you with a quick elevator until you need another lift.

Know this is part of a larger program. Possibly you will introduce the concept of nutrition early and throw small questionnaires and information to test. The more interested they are, the better trained they are. They are possibly trapped at some stage, overwhelmed with fads and other sources of misinformation. When this happens, you will go back to your de-frame tasks to reopen them.

You don't want an external source of nutritional knowledge to impede them. You want to concentrate them on an internal authority. There are two ways to do so, the logical approach and the unconscious approach.

The cognitive approach is a positive one. The distinction between mouth food and stomach food is to be added.

What's food for the mouth? Food in the mouth is a meal that you consume because it tastes amazing. At the moment, you like it. Right now, you're looking for a taste of it. Nutrition from your stomach is nutrition you consume because it gives you strength and makes you feel healthy. In other words, you feel good now when you eat mouth food, but in half an hour, you usually feel bad.

You may or may not care for stomach food now, but you'll be able to eat it in half an hour. You can use hypnotic lightning and a future memory to construct a detailed experience. Weave questions like this into it:

"Is it a mouth food or stomach food any time you talk about food?"

They have to imagine in the future and think about how they feel an hour away to address you. Are they happy they eat everything? Will it makes you feel good or do you feel bad?

If it's a candy bar, have they a sugar crash and guilt? Would they consider that it was enjoyable if it's a salad or something similar? Were they pleased that they had it?

And there may be a time when comfort foods like macaroni and cheese are just what you need. If this is the case, then eat it. Don't take it away. Don't take it away.

You are making them more aware of the Pregnancy Theory system, which is a part of their mind, which monitors nutrition and causes cravings so that nutritional deficiencies can be controlled.

You sensitize them to it with the difference between mouth food and stomach food. It is enough for a lot of men.

Another strategy involves developing a balanced food craving. Individuals are scared of diets because they eat foods they don't want and because they have to give up things they want. But what if you don't give up?

You don't give up if you want something good for you. They just satisfy their appetite. The difference between mouth food and stomach food contributes to the belief that certain good stuff can be craved for you.

What you're doing is essentially making a mental break button, so there's a stage between "have love, eat food." And if you want to enjoy the meal, do so by all means. No big deal. No big deal.

With time, you can turn this into healthy foods. The goal is to encourage them to develop a safe and solid lifestyle.

The simple, direct approach is to build a list of healthy, hypnotically descriptive foods.

The taste of watermelon with wonderful aromas is bursting into your mouth, the salad that just makes you feel refreshed and energy-rich. These are the more straightforward recommendations that work relatively well.

You may prefer a more indirect, unconscious approach. You can do this only by reviving healthier food options when you are searching for something good.

They come home and drink a big glass of water on a hot day, for example, when they are parched. You are telling them:

- "Why have you not been drinking a glass of coke? Why have you not taken a glass of beer?"

- "I just needed a glass of water. After coke, I had it, but the water was the first thing I wanted."

By doing so, you remind them of their good food choice.

When it comes to diet, drinking a lot and plenty of water is a big component. The air is safe. The food is good. It flushes toxins, salts, relieves hunger, and fills the stomach. One of the main things you do will be to help them build a healthy relationship with water. You can use a de-frame test to break it down if they have issues with water. If they believe water is dull, they can enjoy it in different formulations such as teas. Teas and teas can be a beautiful and fairly safe form of drinking water.

Initially, you can revive healthy food choices as a component of stories, since they are prominent. The odds of unexpectedly beginning to live a little better between the sessions are very high. You can start adding identities once you have revived some stories. Which kind of person does this, for example? ... and they begin to live up to that name.

You will then move on to consciousness. In other words, how did you feel like having healthy food and unhealthy food?

In other words, you take the concept of stomach and body food and adapt it to safe and bad cravings. The excessive longing will be a meal for the mouth, and it will be based on an emotional question.

Anything like this is a typical reframe:

- "Have you ever thought of going to the bathroom where you were dead, but you couldn't because people keep watching you"?

And maybe you were thirsty and you were still thirsty, no matter how much water you were drinking in a dream? It never was enough, because your body was thirsty and dreamed water did not quench it, of course. Now the reframe is here. There are other needs that we don't feel fulfilled in the way you think.

If you like a mouth meal, it's never done with a mouth meal. This is an emotional issue. This is accomplished with an emotional approach, where we stick to the emotional aspect of it.

When they develop a repertoire of emotional skills, they handle the emotional drive responsibly and not nutritiously. You teach them to distinguish the difference between the state of mind to a state of mind so that they can recognize that what they want is not a thing dependent on their heads. It is what the body wants. The goal is to develop a desire for nutritious foods. Why? Why? Suppose your body knows what's good for it.

Note that your body enters stress mode when you eat something for which it does not have tolerance. If you can feel this tension consciously or not, the body must know. Yet consciousness itself doesn't even matter.

What matters is this: do their actions fail, and do they make healthy food choices?

In other words, have they a passion for it?

Such cravings can be generated by continually reviving a desire for healthier food choices.

They will always have some form of success between sessions. And if they just make a decent meal in 7 days and loved it, you relive it.

You could only spend half an hour on this success. You could spend 10 minutes on two or three of them for the same result if they have more.

The point is that very few people will be able to make no good food choices. At some point in their lives, nobody wants something healthy, something good for them. It might take some digging, but somewhere it is.

Why is revivification such a useful tool?

And you want to know that the nervous system gets input on positive things. It 's important to have a little healthy awareness, so if they crave candy bars, you know it probably isn't the best thing to revive. You need plenty of dietary awareness if you have a craving for berries, vegetables, meat, and nuts to know these aren't unhealthy per se. You will then revive the desired aspect of it so that it encourages the unconscious to do more.

They are essentially in a craving state without a child's actual conception, weight gain, or illness component of the morning, only the hunger parts, and they begin to crave good things for them.

Another phenomenon that can take place is that when people start eating better as a habit over time when they cut out the healthy part, they feel like something in their lives is lacking. That's the location to which you like them. When people do this randomly, they may fill the missing with an addiction, sugar, or something else that gives them a high level, but that covers the problem.

The way you manage that is by training your attention constantly for a healthy desire, and when you feel the sense of loss, you ask yourself: is it mental, which means you make use of the mental toolkit you gave it?

Nor is it nutritional, in which case what stomach food would fulfill your desire? They make a healthy choice anyway.

4: Your Subject's Self-Image

By self-esteem, we talk of body image in particular. When people have a bad picture of themselves, it feeds back into the emotional part. The bad the body image of someone, the less likely they are to adopt a healthy lifestyle. Why? Why?

There are a few explanations for this. One is embedded in the feeling: "Why bother? My body is ugly, it's awful, it's still my enemy, why should I bother trying to take care of it?"

And then in this kind of thinking, there is ignorance:

"Oh, even I don't know what is happening. I'm so scared of my body, I don't like how it looks, and I don't know, so right now I will go for good and not just good, but in half an hour."

Most positive emotions add up to a very unhealthy lifestyle right now. When someone's view of the body is out of control and seeks to dissociate them from their bodies, the food aspect is less important. Interestingly, they 're not hunting for healthier products, so it just doesn't matter. It's a shame they 're struggling to feel better right now.

Let's now look at someone who has a healthy body and a healthy self-image, spiritual or not.

When they are spiritual, a very simple reframe can be used along the lines:

- "You gave this body some stronger or more strength from above. It's your ride. You may want to know how to care for it."

One sort of reframing is the whole concept that your body is your temple. The notion that their body is their main interface with the world can also act as a legitimate reframe for people who have not been similarly inclined. It's like a connection to the internet. Similar to high-speed broadband, if you have a sluggish dial-up modem, it is easy to say the difference. The same is true for the life experience of your subject.

The more you are in touch with your food and physical needs, the more your brain and mind function, And the greater your life experience.

If you do not have a problem with self-image, you do not have to deal with it. In other words, don't repair it if it's not broken.

One way of finding out whether there is the problem is to ask a set of near-magical questions:

- How do you feel when you look into the mirror?

- Have you ever seen yourself in the mirror of the shower in the nude? Why do you see what you're seeing?

- When you close your eyes and imagine yourself, what do you see at the moment? Describe yourself. Describe yourself.

These questions are almost magical because they evoke an answer. Listen in their descriptions to words and especially adjectives. They are likely to have an issue with their self-image if they use derogatory words such as "horrible, gross, bad, unsafe, nasty." You probably have a good self-image if you use overall compassionate words.

You must always pay attention to your emotional tone and features. The vocabulary may be inherently sympathetic, but if the emotional tone is repulsive, for instance, then a secret decision is probably made. You may be socially friendly by saying what you think you want to hear; however, your feelings will betray you.

How To Help People Improve Their Self-Image

There are two main self-image components. The first is sympathy for oneself, and the second is the prejudice of affirmation. Let's deal with these individuals.

Self-compassion is about being good to you. Knowing you 're good enough, you 're all right. Self-compassion starts where you are from. And if you make poor decisions, you don't want to punish yourself. When you do, cognitive dissonance is formed. Those times you 're not going to want to think about because they feel bad. It means you 're not going to benefit from them, and the chances are high to repeat them. If it gets very bad, you will manifest a part of yourself that binge eats to punish you.

The bad behavior comes out, and you don't control it. This is more like having an alter ego that eats the binge. This is avoided by self-compassion. It helps it to go. You know you made a bad choice of food and binged, but it's all right. Forgive yourself. Forgive yourself. You 're going to do great tomorrow. And that's the next day.

Feeling caring for yourself doesn't mean you let go. This just means that you can make mistakes from time to time. The opposite side is a validation distortion. Whenever you feel bad about your body, you can believe that it is worse than it is. A behavior is: what is the point? You let yourself go, and you become that very thing.

You can hear them say, for example, "Look, I eat well. I am still obese. I'm still overweight. I'm still overweight. I'm still unattractive.

You want to prove yourself correctly. This is the prejudice of belief and one of the psychological effects most difficult to resolve.

Naturally, methods like the classical double-blind language and another mind-altering language can be used.

When a person has an awful self-image, you might ask them:

- "Which body part do you want? Pick just the part of your body that you like even a little.

- "What part of your body would you say is maybe the nicest?

- "How much do people compliment you on what part(s) of your body?

What are they going to say? Who knows? Who knows? Yet something they 're going to have to claim. You will pick one part of your body. You'll assign them a mission then. Suppose your favorite physical feature is your smile. Tell them to note their smile in the following week and then tell you how much they smile.

What you do is continue to use a confirmatory bias to guide you towards the quantities of stuff you like about your body.

It is the old classic Ericksonian double-blind: which one of your hands now feels lighter?

Which one of your hands now feels most unusual?

The fact that they respond means that they are looking for some kind of information. You search for proof.

You may even ask them to remember which part of their body shocked them, so they like it more than they know.

It is the language of mind-bending at work. You 're going to get curious about your body in a way that your connection to your body image searches for things that work.

Let's assume, for starters, that they're overweight. You have other medical conditions as it affects your breathing, your pulse, and your cholesterol levels. No ... they haven't got diabetes. It is really important for the reframe below.

"You tell me that you are putting all this thing in your body and that, as a result, your body has reached that condition, but you have no diabetes. What did your body manage on earth to keep diabetes away while most people have it? This is not a good job. This is a good job. How is your body doing such a good job on earth? This is the secret to self-image to find what they do correctly.

If they're still alive, something's right. If they did anything wrong, they would have another question. They will be dead ... and for that, there's no cure. When you have learned to despise your body early in life, you might continue to relapse and repress.

You can have to make a series of regressions to retrain them to learn how they respond to their bodies. When you like the sound of your voice, you have to know that your body produces the sound.

You can, therefore, thank them. You may revive your singing and your speech and wonder how it is created by your body. And what a wonder your body is. This is a powerful Ericksonian trick that tells them that their bodies are unique. It's an amazing creature. It's an amazing machine that does incredible things. When someone starts appreciating his body as an amazing tool, they 'd like to take better care of it.

Like a guy who loves his car.

They keep it tidy, tidy, and suspicious, particularly with food or drink, when someone comes too close to it. You appreciate that. And what if everyone decided to care about their body in the same way?

People who love their car do not put in cheap fuel or gasoline. It's their kid. It's their kid. I love it. We love it. And they carefully surround it with the finest materials to hold it in top condition. If someone were to relate to their body with the same sensation of wonder as a car enthusiast, they would like to take extra care of it.

It is the core of the process's self-image, to make them enjoy their bodies again, to see the magic of it.

You can do this with basic facts about your body, which contribute to a confirmatory distortion.

You teach a mentality that eventually leads them to believe their body is a wonderful thing worth taking care of.

5. Your Subject's Relationship With Movement

It's about movement, not exercise. Movement is normal, and we all do it every day. If someone thinks about exercising, all kinds of images can be thrown up.

Go to the fitness center. Sweating. Sweating. Acting deliberately in a way that doesn't make you feel better. Perhaps some people are also overwhelmed by the scent of exercise equipment and other people's bodies.

Movement, on the other hand, will probably be something entirely different. Running, Cooking, Yoga, Rollerblading, Baseball.

Look at the difference? Exercise makes some people think of a fitness center. Fitness centers can be intimidating. The more intimidating you are because some of the people who go to the gyms are in fantastic shape! It's a loop of self-fulfillment filled with shame:

"So, I'm overweight and a good little thing in beautiful form over there. I'm feeling bad so that I'm better balanced before I head to the gym."

The other problem is to know what to do when you go to the fitness center. You may be able to learn how to use the equipment safely, but then what? What's a good schedule? How are you waking up? How are you? What good regime? What good regime? Why do you know whether you drive yourself or not? What's the difference between aerobic exercise and strength training, and all that? It's frustrating. It is frustrating.

The argument is that exercise and pain always go hand in hand, while activity means using our physical bodies to do something we enjoy.

Play with children or grandchildren, swim with whales, play sports, if you turn your body, place a strain on your body to the right degree. You don't have to go to the fitness center to do that.

It may be the gym, but there's always an option. Any gesture that is friendly and satisfying would.

This will help them keep their lifestyle safe. So when they eat well and walk around, ultimately, they 're good.

You should try all kinds of activities to find any of them, like boxing or dancing. It not only enhances their health and weight but also raises their quality of life.

In comparison to a system, they have to do as they have a high probability of keeping a system they love. And if the unconscious mind is behind it, it will handle.

The key is to create a protocol or program that someone looks forward to, in fact, to the right lifestyle. You should like to eat, move somewhat, and miss those things if you're deprived of it.

We will feel disappointed and would want to return to it if they are blocked from doing so. As soon as the block disappears, they will automatically return to a healthy lifestyle. This is a method of self-correction. Your goal is to build a lifestyle that presupposes that your weight issue is no longer present. Everything they do with their lives reinforces and reaffirms their health decisions, making them easier to adopt.

How To Encourage and Appreciate Movement

Have you ever been on a long trip, car ride, bus ride, or train journey and have long been confined to your seat?

When you reach your destination, what is the first thing you want to do? You'll typically stand up, shake, stretch, and enjoy moving without any limitations. Yet physical activity, in this case, feels very good.

There are other things that you can do with movement. You may ask them, for example, to remember a time when they felt fantastic while they were dancing or even kicking a ball with their child around the park.

So I would say:

"What if you just felt like shifting your body?"

Then they revive or build a hypnotic stimulus and continue your favorite way of exercising. You may want to go for long walks in the park. Then the hypnotizer produces a potential memory of walking in the park, and as they pass, triggers the anchor, and wow, it feels like walking around.

The argument is that most people can remember a moment when they felt fine about their bodies. Your job is to figure out when it was. The aim is to blend movement with enjoyment and good feelings. Ask people about what form of movement they want. It could be spinning, running, walking the dog, or even kneading the bread during the bakery.

People who move could get out of a station early and walk to the office for an extra block or two. They could take the stairs instead of taking the elevator. These are simple things that can be integrated into your day-to-day routines if you like them.

That's the secret to making it fun. It's not fun to walk up and down the steps. Seek to restore feelings of enjoyment and then move them up the stairs. Make a memory of the future. Pre-live up the steps and feel awesome. Take them to the top of the stairs, thundering with their rhythm, they say:

"I have done it, my Gosh. I feel so good!!"

One of the truths of movement is not overdoing it. Their heartbeat is slightly higher than during usual everyday activities. There is a sweet spot. As soon as their heart rate marginally increases, they are already in the region. They will finally be in their best environment.

Another warning is the burning feeling in the lungs, which means that they lack oxygen and seek to draw even more energy. It is vital, therefore, that your topic isn't too early; otherwise, it will be burned down, and the entire thing will have a negative association. Lung burn does not automatically mean good. Your breath rate should be adequate.

When they find it difficult to talk to anyone, they 're in the field. To most people, a successful goal is to fight a little harder than normal to their air. There is also a rise in body temperature and breathing. They tend to feel warmer and breathe a little heavier.

You may still have a conversation, but a little extra effort might be required. When their breath and temperature are high, their heartbeat is also high. This won't be in a dangerous environment that keeps other people away, but it'll be close.

The benefit of this approach is that they become acclimatized over time to whatever exercise or movement they perform.

They 're no longer going to feel like water. Their respiration will no longer be as busy, so they have to force themselves a little to remain in that environment.

Meanwhile, you continually emphasize the fun aspect of the activity when they come to see you. You increase your body temperature and increase your breathing by adding confirmatory bias.

If walking, running, climbing stairs, ride, swim, dance, football, soccer, tennis ... It doesn't matter. It doesn't matter. As long as their body temperature and breathing increase.

The trick is to find a good balance between where you can't talk and where it's easy to speak.

When their talk begins to work a bit, they 're there. They don't need machinery or technology, because the body knows how they are doing. However, if they're a technology junkie, they can use it by all means. It's going to add value to the entire thing.

Hacks For Weight Loss

You should also inspire your subjects to try out some hacks:

- Take Cold Showers: There are two types of fat in the human body: white and brown. Brown fat appears to be across the neck and chest regions. Whenever these areas get cold, they cause a fat-burning cascade. If someone puts an icepack on their chest or shoulders to cool them, it causes a fat-burning reaction. Often, people who take cold showers or ice baths prefer to slim down because of this.

- Don't Make it Forbidden: Know, it is more attractive if someone rejects. The aim is to cut off candy and treats for your subjects, but occasionally – for example, once a week – they should sleep and eat what they have been resistant to.

This cures the mental burden of avoiding sweets and the like. You don't want to promote excess food – but allow it to be tented once in a while. Moderation is the secret.

Edit your serving plates. Encourage your subjects to buy-side dishes to eat. It is all the food your belly wants. This is a visual thing. It's visual. Upon finishing what is on your plate, you can decide whether to have more. With a larger plate packed with food, eating it is much easier without realizing what you do.

Leave something on their website. You may start with only a few remains and move to the point where they throw away half of their food or save as leftovers. If they are frustrated with throwing away food, the next step is to give them half of the portion, so that they don't waste it. And they will finally develop the habit of consuming a small portion, although it's a bigger plate.

Encourage eating carefully. Tell the subjects to chew as they eat slowly. Get them to know their textures, tastes, and even their food's roots. If they are especially hungry, they can be tempted to hurry, because they can change their knife and bend over to make it harder to eat.

One technique is to use chopsticks – if they are not a professional with them, they would have to eat slowly. Nonetheless, the ultimate aim here is to make them more conscious of the eating process — not only when it comes to what you put in your mouth, but how you do it.

Keep A Journal of Food. This is a great way to track precisely what and how much you consume, particularly in the initial stages, as it illustrates exactly what you put into your body.

There are lots of tips, tricks, and more online hacks. Encourage them to spice up things and shake old habits and feelings.

Last but not least, note that hypnosis is not always a fast cure for weight loss!

You usually have to do at least ten sessions for a subject (although this can vary depending on severity). However, improving their relationship with food, conviction, and motivation to a deep level is suitable for 15 to 30 sessions.

It helps you to deliver a comprehensive package that looks at your whole lifestyle. A whole life that will make them feel better, more involved, happier, and slimmer.

Therefore, the effects last longer than any diet or fad treatment because you have a complete and comprehensive weight loss.

WHY IT REALLY IS HARDER FOR WOMEN TO LOSE WEIGHT

A woman and her husband go together on a diet. Were they inspired both? Yes. Yes. Yes. Should they each count calories faithfully? Sure. Sure. Nonetheless, the man is more likely to lose excess pounds sooner than his partner.

Why? Why? Blame the genes, say some experts.

"There is something that we hear all of the time, and it can be challenging for women," says endocrinologist Ula Abed Alwahab, MD. "And their genetic makeup can sadly make weight loss a little harder for women.

So what factors are at work here?

1. Blues metabolism. In general, women have more body fat and less muscle than men. So it influences the essential metabolic rate or the number of calories the body carries to rest.

"The metabolic rate is partly determined by the muscle mass, and women have less fat and muscle than men," Dawn Noe, a nutritionist and educator of diabetes, said.

2. Effects of pregnancy. When a woman is pregnant, her weight and body fat increase. Moreover, a new mother also finds it difficult to sleep and exercise. And both of them will need to lose those additional pounds.

Nevertheless, at this stage of life, breastfeeding helps with losing calories and weight loss.

3. Menopause. Women often gain weight during menopause by loss of estrogen and slower metabolism in their abdomen. Some women also have a name for their new vase —

Mesopotamia.

4. PCOS struggles. About 5 and 10% of women suffer from polycystic ovary syndrome (PCOS). This is characterized by a hormonal imbalance, which makes a loss of weight harder and makes menstrual irregularity more difficult.

Notwithstanding these challenges, weight gain, and succeed in several ways. There are three of them here.

1. Include resistance and weight training.

Muscle building helps both men and women improve their metabolism. Additional muscle mass lets you lose calories even when you sit down or rest.

You should preserve your muscle by resistance exercises for 20 to 30 minutes per session at least twice a week. It is especially important when you get older. (Your metabolism slows down naturally, so you lose your muscle as you grow old.)

Many ways to approach resistance training are available:

- Using equipment in the fitness center or the house.

- Using free weights or bands of resistance.

- Take part in a workout party, such as Pilates.

- Use the body with push-ups, squats, and lunges for resistance.

Women often refuse to do weight training because they believe that they would look manly. It is a myth, though, since women lack the testosterone they have in men.

Noe allows women to weigh comfortably. "Women should undergo weight training to achieve muscle-building benefits such as higher metabolic rate and osteoporosis prevention," She said.

Bearing weight exercise isn't just safe since weight-bearing exercise is preparation. As it helps you grow in muscle mass, you eat more calories, which greatly reduces insulin resistance and helps prevent diabetes.

2. Find the eating pattern that works best for you.

When both a middle-aged man and a woman want to lose weight, the calories that a man requires for weight loss are around 1.500 each day (according to the physical activity height/weight/level), but the calorie requirements for a woman are much reduced – usually around 1.200 calories per day, says Noe.

Of course, both of these calories will move slightly higher if they exercise frequently. To keep weight loss for women can mean eating less than men in the long term.

A balanced food scheme like the Mediterranean diet is often recommended by Noe. It also tends to use lower carbohydrates and ketogenic diets, particularly for women with PCOS or diabetes who can not support higher carbohydrate meal plans. "Weight loss research does not indicate one diet pattern over another," she says, "and the diet pattern which you select must be tailored to your health needs and eating behaviors."

3. Focus on the long game.

Being patient is necessary. Research indicates that the majority of weight loss programs will result in weight losses of 5 % to 10% within one year. "Talk with your healthcare team if you do not see success, and you might need to seek out a new program that suits your lifestyle better," she says.

If you adopt a fat-free, low-carbon diet or some other diet, make sure that your meals are healthy and nutritious. Include lean proteins as well as good fats such as pasta, olive oil and avocados, minimal single carbohydrates (no sugar, white bread, cakes), and plenty of vegetable and fruit minerals.

For women over the age of 50, other nutrition recommendations include maintaining appropriate calcium and vitamin D, both from foods or supplements.

WEIGHT LOSS HYPNOSIS IS NOT A MAGIC WAND

Multiple factors cause weight gain. If you look for the reasons, you will deal with emotional problems, how to deal with stress by eating comfort, food selection, and a sedentary lifestyle. All three of these factors contribute to excess weight accumulation. Many people are overweight due to the way they handle stress. Emotional eating is one of the main factors that prevent a person from maintaining the ideal weight.

There are several approaches to deal with problems, and hypnotherapy is one of the solutions.

Some Figures about Obesity

According to the Health and Social Care Information Center, in 2011, the balanced body mass index (BMI) was just 34% of men and 39% of women. The ideal BMI is described as a figure from 18.5 to 25.

The National Health Service provides some other troubling figures:

- 24% of men in the UK in 2011 were obese. In contrast, the figure for obesity was 13 percent in 1993.

- In 2011, 26 percent of women were obese, compared to 16 percent in 1993.

- 9.5 percent of all children 4 to 5 years of age were obese.

- Almost 53% of men and 44% of women were

overweight, with high blood pressure in 2011.

- There were 11,736 hospital admissions due to medical obesity-related issues.

Emotional Issues

Most people believe they should just eat, and the excess weight will vanish. Diets typically fail because of emotional eating and other psychological issues, which must first be resolved for a positive result.

According to psychologists, most overweight people try to cope with a certain emotional problem. Stress, financial problems, problems with relationships, and lack of adequate sleep may all lead to this.

Weight loss starts with a change in your beliefs and emotions. Hypnosis can help a lot here. Nevertheless, hypnosis can in no way be viewed as a magic curtain. A concerted effort is needed to bring about improvement in your life.

Choosing the Right Diet

The first move is to deal with emotional issues. Choosing intelligent foods is just as important. There's no need to feed yourself. Fad diets are ineffective. Typically, the dietary habits and foods you consume will change. Healthy snacks help regulate cravings and weight loss.

Some foods must be avoided by all people irrespective of attempts to lose weight. Both hydrogenated oils, huge amounts of salt, refined sugars, and human-made sweeteners should be avoided.

Be More Active

A sedentary lifestyle is a major issue for many people who work in an office and feel incredibly exhausted at home. Nevertheless, there are ways to stay healthy without going to the gym every day.

Speedy walks, walking with your kids in the park, and ascending the stairs rather than using the elevator are improvements in the right direction. You must be serious about weight loss and do it for yourself. Determining and visualizing will motivate you. Professional help such as hypnotherapy can also make the process easier.

IS SELF HYPNOSIS WEIGHT LOSS RIGHT FOR YOU?

Self-hypnosis is an effective approach for women to lose weight in very special circumstances. There will be a variety of questions when determining if this strategy will be used for weight loss. Who can I trust, how long will it take, hypnotics alone will do the trick? While many promoters of audio and videotapes represent rapid self-hypnosis weight loss, it is important to distinguish between those who offer a broader weight loss regime and not simply rely on self-hypnosis as an instant healing procedure. Research by Vanderbilt University criticized most self-hypnosis weight loss methods on the internet; however, it found that some pages offered what appeared to be legitimate self-hypnosis weight loss programs.

Here we provide you with valuable knowledge to make informed decisions as to whether you use self-hypnosis as a way to minimize your weight or whether diets and drugs have not worked for you or whether you find self-hypnosis as your primary attempt to lose weight. The good news is that weight loss through self-hypnosis is generally considered safe if someone qualified for training in these techniques has properly trained and advised you. Besides, the cost of this type of weight loss is normally lower than many other choices if you do not need an additional technique to achieve your objective in your particular case. Nonetheless, most individuals may need one or more additional strategies, for example, exercise and nutritional therapy. If you want a fast fix, other options are available, but they are much more expensive, including loss of weight of Bariatric.

There is a range of organizations that offer clinical monitoring and credential requirements that help uphold hypnotherapy standards and ethics. The American Council of Hypnotherapy Examiners may also be the group that is mostly dedicated to certifying hypnotherapy colleges. Another association, founded by the National Board of Certified Clinical Hypnotherapists in the 1990s, created a certification framework for practitioners to set up guidelines for the hypnosis field. The National Council for Licensed Clinical Therapists defines itself as 'an educational, scientific and professional hypnotherapist organization which promotes public and professional knowledge of the benefits of hypnotherapy and supports scientific research into the uses of hypnotherapy.'

While the hypnosis practitioner is significantly confirmed, it is not always foolish evidence or the only deciding factor when it comes to self-hypnosis. As in the medical field, doctors are not certified by the board in their specific medical sector but are non-incompetent and can serve their patients well. It is advisable to check if there are any reports or references which require independent verification of the skills of the practitioner. Finally, consider claims that seem too good to be true and whether other options may be more suitable for you, depending on your circumstances, such as bariatric weight loss, which we provide with further information as an alternative self-hypnosis weight loss.

SELF-HYPNOSIS HELPS PCOS WEIGHT LOSS EFFORTS IN WOMEN

Most PCOS women can solve much of their health issues by losing only 7% to 10% of their body weight. Nevertheless, the metabolic nature of PCOS can lead to a loss of weight. Some studies indicate that women with PCOS have to work 25 percent harder than lean women to use the same amount of stored fat as energy. Home self-hypnosis is an important method that women with PCOS may use to achieve significant weight loss.

Self-hypnosis is a way to rapidly and effectively understand new behaviors. Weight loss and, above all, keeping it off, calls for developing new behaviors. Self-hypnosis is a healthy and fun way to improve your learning. It allows you to see immediate outcomes, which increase your interest in learning more. It turns out that what you spend your time doing has a strong effect on what you do and what you do. What you expect would have a lot of effect on what you encounter.

Ninety percent of people losing weight recover, plus more-the numbers are well-known to dietary people for life and are expected of us, ninety percent. When you are willing to lose weight (again and again), encouraging your efforts in self-hypnosis may be the secret to lifelong success.

There is a group of people who lose substantial weight and never recover. 10% are people who have learned how to sustain a substantial loss of weight for years. They share other characteristics:

They 're all eating less than fat;

They all practice regularly and most days average an hour of activity.

They all keep a close eye on the scales and check the truth regularly.

Hypnosis, or, in particular, self-hypnotization, can help you to learn this behavior, and also ENJOY. The first two behaviors show the common sense 'just eat well and exercise' which frustrated millions who regularly try not to do this. The third item, the daily scale-checking fact, suggests the secret to breaking a cycle to failure the plagues most dietitians.

Careful people learn to connect the dots. "If I do so, I get similar results; I get different results when I do so." Keeping a close eye on your bathroom scale, as you lose weight and particularly when you move to a healthier lifelong diet, will improve the insight you have about what behaviors are getting you results. Health research explores how our perceptions and attitudes are formed. "To research cognition is important the notion that beliefs can be distorted with expectations," said Michael I. Posner, an emeritus neuroscience professor at the University of Oregon and a specialist in attention. "But, we get to the processes now."

Hypnosis is a method of deep relaxation that significantly increases the ability to think. It is a powerful and potentially misuse operation. On the other hand, self-hypnosis is a wonderful device that you manage for your own best interests.

The recent studies of the brain activity of hypnosis prone people indicate that their brains have significant improvements in the way they interpret knowledge as they act on suggestions during hypnosis. The changes fundamentally change how people see, feel, hear, taste, and interact with what is real. Hypnosis can alter the perception of the reality of an individual. So, standing on the scale and looking out for 150 pounds and thinking, "I'm fat! " you teach yourself, and you think you 're a fat man. Seeing the 150 on your scale and thinking, "I am a person losing fat," you are more likely to think this (especially when you saw 154 a week ago) and to behave like a person who loses weight. And then, that's what you do.

Hypnosis was well-known for dubious entertainment. A hypnotizer allows a participant to trance or relax and implies that a hypnotized person may provide clarification of what is real. When you say that you're like a chicken – if you're able to click on the stage at any point, you'll entertain the audience with chicken behaviors. The suggestion that you do so accidentally is at issue. There is no proof that a hypnotized person behaves in ways that contradict his or her beliefs or will. But if you are ready to be an entertainer (take a stage, as any unhypnotized volunteer does), then you'll be able to click once, if this is the entertainment you suggest.

Although it does little work, hypnosis has been used in medicine since the 1950s to treat pain, and more recently to treat anxiety, depression, trauma, irritable bowel syndrome, and food disorders. Throughout India, physicians used hypnosis effectively as anesthesia also for limb amputation in the 19th century. Hypnosis was no longer used until ether became available.

Brain experts also don't know exactly what the hypnotic state is. This could just be a normal type of deep focus in which you avoid stimuli in the room while concentrating on your thoughts. Recent work on hypnosis and feedback also offers new insight into the learning process and normal functioning of the brain, according to Dr. Posner and others.

It shows that information from the eyes, ears, and body is transferred to primary sensory areas of the brain. This travels from there to other places where understanding takes place. For example, a light that bounces off a rose first enters the eye and becomes a pattern that is sent into the visual center of the brain. There is an appreciation of the rough form of the rose. This pattern is then sent to the next functional area, where color is defined, and then to the next area, where the shape and color are added to create the rose image, together with any other rose information that you have gathered.

They view sounds, fragrances, touches, and other sensory details in the same way. This direction of flow is called feedforward by researchers. As raw sensory information is converted to a pleasant feeling in bundles of nerve fibers, the data is transported from the ground upward.

The surprise is the amount of traffic that is called feedback from top to bottom. There are ten times as many nerve fibers that carry information as they carry it up.

Such complex input routes mean that consciousness is based on what brain scientists term "top-down processing," which ensures that what people see, hear, understand, and believe. What you see isn't necessarily what you get, because what you see depends on the context. You use what you already know to help you understand the raw material-a rose or a hammer is shown. 150 is a number that means effectively "fat" or "weight loss."

This brain structure demonstrates hypnosis, which is so effective top-down that the hypnotic suggestions that you make yourself become a reality. Brain tests indicate that your connection to facts that you have come to know is altered by hypnosis. "I still gain weight" or "I can never lose this overweight." can be replaced with "I'm losing weight effectively" and "I'm losing weight."

When you want to lose weight and keep it off, you can use self-hypnosis to transform how you think about yourself and what you are capable of. Once you do so, you can find yourself behaving in ways that make your dream image possible. Imagine being able to serve yourself happily each day in a certain way.

WEIGHT LOSS TIPS FROM WOMEN WHO HAVE LOST 100 POUNDS

It is a super personal thing to decide to lose weight. And if you never feel you need, it's up to you if you WANT to start a weight loss journey. The thing is, weight loss, especially a large amount — can't be a pill or a tea or shake. Although companies may try to sell you, long-term changes in lifestyles (not a costly meal-replacement shake) take place to make a solid difference.

That could contribute to more nutritionally dense foods being added, sleep as a priority, stress management in a healthy way, and maybe even some physical exercise. This should be something that you can manage for the long term, regardless of your approach.

When you want to excel in weight loss, you must focus more on just how you look. An approach that takes your feelings, your overall health, and mental health into account are often the most effective.

As no two weight loss journeys are the same, we asked a group of women who undertook a big weight loss, just like they did.

A. Gessi Parisi-Rodriguez, 25 Years Of Age, Alexandria, Virginia
Total weight loss: 124 pounds

Start in your comfort zone: Parisi-Rodriguez started her fitness journey with one foot on the other. "When I weighed 252 pounds, I was terrified about going into the gym and working out. I began walking around my block rather—which I was already comfortable with." She worked her way from 30 minutes to two hours' walks, lacing up five or six times a week.

Stop soda. Stop soda. "I have been addicted for years to Pepsi and Dr. Pepper," said Parisi-Rodriguez, who used to drink up to six cans a day. "When I realized that soda was nothing other than empty calories, I swapped my drink instead of water. At first, it was super awkward, but eight years later, I can honestly say I don't want soda any more as I did before.

Lighten up carbohydrates — not digging them. Carbs had long been a key element in the life of Parisi-Rodriguez, born into a family of chefs, pizza makers, and restaurant owners. Instead of giving up carbs — as though! — she reached staples such as bread and tortillas for low-calorie or low-carb versions.

Cancel the whole thing of "all-or-nothing." "I used to think that I was losing everything that day if I ate healthy all day, but then 'slipped up' by eating a cookie," says Parisi-Rodriguez. "So I will just keep binge-eating crap out of it all! "The reframing of her thought allows her to proceed without remorse or deprivation.

From the rooftops, shout your target. Parisi-Rodriguez began to document her progress on Instagram at the onset of her weight loss journey. "This helped to keep me accountable because I knew other people were watching," she says, adding that individuals can also do so by communicating with only another person.

B. Alex Wittner, 23 Years Of Age, Sarasota, Florida
Total weight loss: 105 pounds

Pound that water. Pound the water. 'I still bring a 32-ounce water bottle,' says Wittner, who does not fill this baby once, twice, but four times a day.

Freebies Score fitness class. Wittner also found that a lot of local studios offer free trials and super discounted rates for newbies as a big fan of ClassPass. "Please take advantage of it! The worst thing that can happen is you didn't like it, and you wasted an hour, "she says.

Don't worry about the weight room. For its results, Wittner credits WW (formerly Weight Watchers) and Weight Lifting. "Lifting weights greatly helped me to tone up and lose weight," she says. Although she has learned how to pump iron in a local gym, she goes to YouTube and Insta, where free tutorials are available.

Eat lunch. Serve dinner. And ice cream! Ice cream!

"Deprivation will just take you later off the road," she says. "Not only can I have these now and then, but I'm making healthier homemade versions like a pita pizza or a protein shake which tastes like ice cream."

C. Shannon Mcdaniel-Posey, 32 Years Of Age, Slidell, Louisiana
Total weight lost: 120 pounds in 16 months
Want it — for enhancement. "You need to be conscious," says McDaniel-Posey, who had a wake-up call after the death of her grandfather about her poor physical and mental fitness. "Whatever I wanted, I ate and drank and lost myself. I've been fulfilled to live my life like I was.

Give yourself a break from GD. "A bad meal isn't going to make you fat," she says. "Life is too short of beating you."

Using Facebook. Using Snapchat. "On so many ways it affected me," she says. "There were people like myself who shared photos, recipes, loved products, foodstuff shops, trials and tribulations, and their lives in general. It's been uplifting! It was the motivation that I sought.

D. Tanque Johnson, 26 Years Of Age, New Jersey
Total weight loss: 135 pounds
Cancel the whole, "but I need a coach! "Story, story. "Simple excuses," Johnson says. "I never had a nutritionist or trainer, but knowing what I needed to be helped me remain focused, and my lifestyle changed for the better."

Learn the easiest meal math in the world. Protein (like chicken) + veggies (almost green) = supper is served. Johnson says adding more meats and vegetables to her plate helped her minimize the number of calories she consumed. "It is not a matter of taking carbs from your diet, but acknowledging that they are not necessary at every meal."

E. Jessica Beniquez, 24 Years Of Age, Tampa, Florida
Total weight lost: More than 170
Water Sparkling + Crystal Light = soda who!? Since leaving

carbonated BEVs in the Cold Turkish isn't always easy, this cocktail will help you move, says Beniquez. If she still craves a sweetened drink, she sips this combination.

Get all up in the candy of nature. At night, Beniquez switches sucrose fruit treats. Recall fruit? It's really sweet and hits the place.

"Routine shouting" repeat after me. Once Benique reaches a plateau of weight loss, she changed gears completely. "I've adjusted my eating routine or the way I worked out," she says. "I instead reflect on why I started and how far I would go if I didn't give up."

F. Mayra Arias, 35 Years Of Age, Laguna Beach, California
Total weight loss: 135 pounds
Cook food worth a week in one go. "It's the easiest way to keep track," says Arias. "I didn't have any excuses because I had food ready to heat up." Some of her favorites included the egg roll in a saucepan, Alfredo chicken broccoli, veggie salmon with a saucepan, and parmesan chicken.

G. Suzanne Ryan, 35 Years Of Age, San Francisco Bay Area, California
Total weight loss: 120 pounds
Build trust with baby steps. "A small step has led to some major changes and trust in my ability to stick to something," Ryan made the first move: swapping soda for flat or sparkling water. "Simple changes can lead to big results – so start with one thing if you feel overwhelmed, then add."

Stay in your lane. Stay in your lane. "Do what works for you, don't compare with others," she says. "Everyone is different, and there is no single-size approach."

H. Shanna Fichera, 31 Years Of Age, Camarillo, California
Total weight loss: 110 pounds
Start small. Start small. "Fifteen minutes a day, I started to walk or jog. I worked up to thirty, then increased it again. This

was a very positive process."

Don't give up the plateaus for weight loss. "I recall hitting and feeling so discouraged on the first plateau, but you have to get through and keep putting in the effort to get your plan going.

I. Brianna Blank, 22 Years Of Age, Westbrook, Connecticut
Total weight loss: 150 pounds

Find your favorite healthy meal and eat it all the time. "I looked at the food available in the restaurant to find the healthiest choices at college and sat on a turkey sandwich with all-wheat bread and mustard. I was so determined to meet my goals that it did not feel boring."

J. Maria Gordon, 31 Years Of Age, Upper Marlboro, Maryland
Total weight loss: 104 pounds

Start with a little adjustment. "I realized I drank a lot of sugar and calories, so I challenged myself only to drink water for 30 days.

Make healthier your old favorites. "I have always loved burgers and fries, and I have started creating healthy food variants, such as turkey burgers with wheat bread and pommy fries."

Get ready for heavy food. "If I know I'm going to dinner, probably want to eat extra calories, all day, I'm eating smaller meals, like breakfast smoothie and lunch salad."

K. Alyssa Ann Heidemann, 34 Years Of Age, Sioux Falls, South Dakota
Total weight loss: 131 pounds

Swap foods that are not helping you. 'I used to eat chips, sweets, and other processed foods all day long, but now I [make more nutritious choices] six times a day. My new snacks include protein bars or shakes, pistachios, PB2 celery sticks (lower fat peanut butter), and low-fat stringed cheese.''

Take vegetables if you are uncomfortable with a meal or snack. "If I'm still hungry, rather than junk food, I turn to vegetables."

Load snacks at work for late nights. "My weakness was fast food on my way home from work at 9:30 to 10 p.m. I now bring food and snacks to my work, so I don't miss and feel more in control when I go home."

Say no to recharges. "I had been drinking diet daily, and I was popping daily. When restaurants gave me refill after refill, I was going to lose track of how much I drank.

L. Sara Lugger, 39 Years Of Age, Oxford, Michigan
Total weight loss: 149 pounds

During your lunch break, move around. "I'll walk on the treadmill at work or outside for 30 to 40 minutes during my lunch."

Everywhere, stash snacks. "I am keeping protein bars in my bag and car. I fend off malnutrition, so I don't eat overeat later."

Eat more often. Eat more often. "I went to six small meals a day for three meals a day."

Split meals with a friend in the restaurant. "I finish eating smaller portions when I share meals without being tented by leftovers on my plates. If I don't have any person to split meals, I put half the portion into a pickup box immediately."

M. Stephanie Aromando, 31 Years Of Age, Sandyston, New Jersey
Total weight loss: ~100 pounds

Shift weights to weight reduction. "While cardio helped me burn fat, powerlifting played a big role in my success. Lifting heavy weights with a trainer helped me to sculpt my body. I was able to squat with 360 pounds after some four months of training—25 more than I had weighed when I started my loss journey."

Always move, even for days of rest. "I work six days a week and go hiking or yoga school once a week on an optional rest day."

Keep it easy. Keep it plain. "I take a minimalist diet approach: my food plan is made from leans (chicken breast, white eggs, and ground turkey), complex carbohydrates (quinoa, sweet potatoes, oatmeal), good fats (coconut oil, almond, avocado) and leafy, grassy green vegetables.

Shop the grocery store's perimeter. "All I need is in a product section, meat storage, or dairy section. I avoid the food center aisles without searching for specific pantry items, such as quinoa or oatmeal."

Prepare food beforehand. "I eat five small meals a day, but only make them in large lots twice a week so that when I'm hungry, all is done and prepared to go."

Drink all the tea. Drink all the tea. "The whole day, I carry a gallon of water with myself until it is over. It looks ridiculous to drag it around the campus, but I don't care."

N. Tanisha Shanee Williams, 33 Years Of Age, Brooklyn, New York

Total weight loss: 140 pounds

When you don't feel like you go to the gym, put on music. "To be healthy physically is nothing that needs to go to the gym, but it's necessary to move your body and burn your calories. I just put my music on when I don't want to go and either dance or hula hoop with my niece."

O. Jade Scooby, 28 Years Of Age, Bangor, Maine
Total weight loss: 140 pounds

Choose a physical activity that you enjoy. "Cardio bores me so much. Powerlifting has changed and saved my life."

Use your advantage with tech and other tools. "I only began by cutting small stuff like soda out one by one, so I wouldn't give up myself mentally. I found myself counting calories on MyFitnessPal, [a huge help] in my weight loss for me. I lost my way a little bit several years ago, and found Renaissance Diet templates that helped me rebuild a healthy relationship with food."

Feed each meal with a combination of carbs and protein. "[I began to track macros [fat, protein, and carbs] when I started counting calories], and I started changing my body even more for the better."

A NEW MOTHER'S GUIDE TO WEIGHT LOSS - PREGNANCY POUNDS CAN BE SHED QUICKLY WITH HYPNOSIS

Bringing a child into the world can make you very happy. This motherhood phase is perhaps one of the best moments for a woman. However, the results are not the same, especially if you want to go back to your previous form and lose weight. How can you find the time to get rid of the weight you gained during your pregnancy with a new baby?

You may consider diets and workouts, but you are likely limited in time because the baby is your priority. Besides, enormous efforts are needed to get through it. As this is the problem for most women who wish to lose pregnancy-related weight, they need to be offered clear weight loss programs.

Luckily, some of the weight gained during pregnancy was shown to decrease through hypnosis. It acts much like treatment so that in a matter of weeks, you can lose weight without having to struggle too hard. Not only that, but you can also relax and decrease the tension in your body due to all the stress.

With hypnosis, you can devote more time to your baby rather than in the gym. There's no need to think about what food you can eat. It is because hypnosis allows you to select the best food without knowing you are deprived. Hypnosis can potentially be a healthy weight loss device.

Hypnosis can also motivate you to combat impulsive food, which is one of the triggers for weight gain. It can be stressful to maintain your weight, particularly when you have to reduce your appetite. You won't have to suffer under hypnosis, with the advantage of losing weight on the way.

If you are worried about increasing numbers because of

pregnancy on the weighing scale display, there is no need to worry. Returning to form will not be a problem with hypnosis. With this approach, you can now lose your pregnancy and spend more precious moments with your newborn boy.

HOW TO REPROGRAM YOUR MIND TO EAT LESS AND ENJOY FOOD MORE

Every action we take has an underlying motivation.

You will figure out how to reprogram the mind to eat less and to enjoy food more, by understanding the influence of discomfort and enjoyment (or neuro-associations) in every decision and action. This is an important piece of the puzzle about weight loss that I hope will help you to understand why you struggled to lose weight and to keep it hidden in the past.

Maybe we don't think about it, but the unconscious part of our mind is the engine behind our thoughts and conducts. For example, you may want to lose weight for a long time, but have continued to put it off or said: "I will begin next week." You know that you want to become better, so that's how you go about it. This is because you deliberately associate more pain with intervention than you do with the postponement.

I bet you slim down for your wedding or other important days, but you had more discomfort than your diet, but you didn't look good on your special day. In this situation, you have changed what you associated with pain. Any move and adaptation to your preferred equipment were even more difficult than adhering to this strict weight loss program.

Once we hit a point of suffering for which we are unable to recover, something changes inside us.

The major issue is that most of us determine what pain or enjoyment is associated with the short term and not in the long term. This is why it is so much easier to enjoy this second dessert aid because now you can taste pleasure. Although that pleasure is not too indulgent, a beautiful body, at that moment, is something too abstract and so the mind drives for the immediate gratification. To obtain long-term pleasure, we need to learn to break the wall of short-term pain. It is a critical issue. If we learn how the mind works, we can build instruments and skills that can benefit us.

It's important to realize here that it isn't pain that pushes us, but the belief that anything contributes to pain. Likewise, the confidence that anything that contributes to happiness is not a true pleasure. This is a very critical distinction. It is not the reality that drives us, but our false conceptions of reality. When you do not take steps, you can be sure that there is one reason: you have learned to mix more pain than not.

There is only only one path to change: to change what you are linking pain and pleasure. You may make a short-term adjustment otherwise, but it will not last, so you know. You had a diet before, and you wanted to force yourself and discipline, but as long as you had the discomfort of consuming the foods that helped you, it was doomed to fail because we were programmed to strive for the idea of pleasure.

Strength is not enough to alter what you identify unconsciously. The good news is that we can actively change our minds in conjunction with pain and pleasure. This is a great aspect of changing your relationship to food – change your behavior by linking pain and pleasure to you.

Let's take a step further with the idea of positive, pleasurable, and negative, painful associations. I'm sure you want to finish a portion of everything in general. A chocolate bar, a packet of snacks, or anything on your plate. This was not long ago that food shortages were widespread, and we can combine satisfaction with what is before us. So, unconsciously and possibly consciously, if I asked you not to finish a portion, you feel that you deny yourself.

Your brain constantly processes what your senses experience and creates a dynamic network of unconscious interconnections between thoughts, images, sonorities, and feelings. If you feel severe pain emotionally or physically, the brain looks for a source immediately. When the cause is found by your brain, it links the connection in your nervous system to make you feel the pain again in the future. This is an alert signal that when you get into a situation like this, you should check. This also helps you in learning what to do so that you can return to friendly states and do so more easily than without the program. It is our instinct for survival at work.

It is time to recondition your mind and feelings to associate discomfort with unhealthy food and to connect pleasure with the thought of consuming healthy foods and smaller amounts.

Associating satisfaction with healthy eating and knowing when your belly feels full is an important factor in weight loss. You will make yourself content to not finish something by manipulating your mind and by mixing gratification to drive away from the plate while it is still fed. And just eat half the sandwich and leave half the broth. This may sound wasteful, I realize, but you can still feed your pets, save them for lunch tomorrow or freeze them again.

Action: Change What You Link Pain And Pleasure To.
How do you link pleasure to the action of eating less?

Step 1: An apple, a candy bar, a croissant, a slice of pasta and breakfast, lunch and dinner are available each day, and half of the food can be divided, and you can see precisely how much a half slice is.

Step 2: If you have achieved your target number, move away from the food, and instantly establish a mental condition of good feelings by actively remembering your positive behavior towards your goal.

Step 3: Think of yourself as an ideal image and make the connection between not finishing everything on your plate and achieving your target.

Step 4: Play a song you like, or you choose a mantra that motivates you to do exactly half what you eat every time you finish. Combine the positive feelings of a song or mantra with the operation to leave the food behind.

It is crucial that you become optimistic, excited, and feel the positive feeling of joy in this achievement and the anticipation of achieving your goal.

Step 5: Repeat this process over and over until you find that you eat something automatically.

You will finally find that you will start pushing your plate away without even noticing it! Do you believe that this would be a liberating experience? To be safe when you eat whatever you want, but to know and understand that you should eat the right amount. In this way, you consciously strengthen the idea that less is more, and you make the mind more moderate.

Remember:

- Do not complete this section and combine the joy of leaving any behind.

- Do this every time you eat, and whilst it is challenging at first, you will find that it will be automatic over a few weeks. It's such a liberating feeling.

- When it comes to food, feel the sense of empowerment and pleasure of action, eat what you want but eat moderately instead of feeling like you negate something.

HOW YOU CAN REDUCE YOUR CORTISOL LEVELS TO REDUCE YOUR WEIGHT

What Is Cortisol?

Cortisol is the main stress hormone of your body. If you are blurry or frightened, the adrenal glands pump it out. This is why we know cortisol best to fuel the "fight or flight" reflex of your body. Do you always feel uneasy after a close call while on the highway, or are you alarmed in the morning? At the function, that's cortisol.

Cortisol plays an important role in our lives, though we most frequently equate this hormone with bad things. Most cortisol is good for the body as it has anti-inflammatory properties and needs to act optimally in our bodies.

If a person is depressed, the surrenal drugs release cortisol from the steroid hormone.

Cortisol is the key stress hormone of the body and plays a part in many body functions, including the blood sugar balance. The blood level of cortisol is normally higher in the morning and decreases slowly during the day.

Cortisol also plays a role in:

- Control of sleep-wake cycles of the body

- Controlling how carbohydrates, fats, and proteins are used in the body

- Reduction of infection

- Blood pressure regulation

Why is higher cortisol an issue?

To release the right amount of cortisol, the body relies on efficient contact between the following three parts:

- the pituitary gland

- the adrenal gland

- the hypothalamus, which is part of the brain

Between them, cortisol is stimulated when the body needs it and blocked when the levels have to fall backward. Too much and too little cortisol may have a detrimental effect on the body.

High cortisol level symptoms

Excess cortisol may be caused by a tumor or by certain drugs. Too much cortisol may contribute to the syndrome of Cushing. Symptoms are as follows:

- frequently

- decreased sex drive

- changes in mood, such as feeling irritable or low

- rapid weight gain in the face and abdomen

- high blood pressure

- a flushed face

- muscle weakness

- increased thirst

- urinating more

- osteoporosis

- bruises or purple stretch marks appearing on the skin

Many people may also consider their cycles to belong or to end.

So much cortisol can also cause other symptoms and disorders, including:

- impaired brain function

- type 2 diabetes

- fatigue

- high blood pressure

- infections

Low Cortisol Level Symptoms

Too little cortisol may cause the disease of Addison. Symptoms include This condition:

- gradual weight loss

- areas of the skin turning darker

- changes in mood

- dizziness

- muscle weakness

- fatigue

- low blood pressure

How To Lower Cortisol Levels Naturally

The good news is ten obvious ways – like dietary adjustments and lifestyle improvements – to raising the cortisol levels.

1. Cut Out Caffeine, Or Consume Less

A 2005 research in the journal Psychosomatic Medicine found that caffeine increases the secretion of cortisol even in sleeping people. As caffeine can boost blood pressure and cortisol production, Krista King, MS, RDN, from Composed Nutrition, offers a solution for lower cortisol: "Try to re-install caffeine. Decrease each day the quantity of caffeine by swapping it for an alternate caffeine-free or lower caffeine."

2. Reduce Your Sugar Intake

If you are looking to reduce the cortisol levels, you will avoid foods that have been heavily processed and pumped full of added chemicals and sugars. "Simple sugars should be reduced (or removed) as one way of combating elevated cortisol levels, pressures, and weight gains," says Balk. The key foods in this group of high sugars include:

- pastries

- candies

- white bread

- cakes

- sodas

Although these hints may give you a temporary boost in energy (and the inevitable boost of cortisol), Balk recommends concentrating on other energy sources. "Because your body needs to receive sugar still to fuel itself, focus instead of simple sugars on having complex carbohydrates." Jim White RD, ACSM, and Jim White Fitness and Nutrition Studios owner also add that fiber-rich foods, protein, and healthy fats help maintain normal cortisol content.

Stress-reducing foods and lower cortisol include:

- fruit

- dairy products

- whole grains (like a bowl of oatmeal with a banana and almond butter)

- starchy vegetables (potatoes, corn, peas

- protein foods (like scrambled eggs with spinach)

3. Avoid Or Limit Alcohol Intake When You're Stressed.

Because alcohol often makes people feel easy and relaxed, you might think it can reduce cortisol levels. The exact opposite is true. Research published in The Journal of Clinical Endocrinology & Metabolism found that people who only have one drink a week have seen their cortisol levels increase by three percent and can be even higher if you are pressurized.

"We see people who drink alcohol to help relax, but alcohol is a depressant and, while you can feel 'better' at present, alcohol is causing several problems that come later," said Amanda A. Kostro Miller, RD, Smart Healthy Living Advisory Board.

"Alcohol can also worsen your mood. Couple depressive moods with stress (or depression), and maybe you're in a terrible rut," she says. "Alcohol will interrupt deep sleep too, so you can not only feel hunger after a drinking night but also feel sick and lose a good night's sleep!"

4. Stay Hydrated

"To drink the water your body needs every day will increase your body's cortisol balance," says White. "The exhaustion in our body can be used as a stressor in the body that can affect the cortisol levels."

A 2018 study conducted by young soccer players shows that even mild dehydration can raise cortisol levels. In other words, don't be afraid of a little H2O if you want to keep your cortisol levels at bay.

5. Stick To A Regular Eating Schedule

Although sometimes difficult, it is a good way to keep stress under control (that darn cortisol trigger). It is partially because it takes the uncertainty where the next meal will be, which in itself may be a source of anxiety. On the other side, keeping to a schedule may also help to avoid stress eating, a new habit which can lead to cortisol levels, particularly when we tend to hit sweets and comfort foods that raise cortisol when overwhelmed.

"Recognize if and when you eat stress: consider maintaining a daily eating routine so you can never get too hungry and stop starving yourself to the max," Miller suggests. "Take a moment before you catch a snack to ask yourself if you're really hungry. You might think you are stressed and looking for something or bored with it. Try to structure a meal-and-snack routine every 3-4 hours while you're awake."

6. Pinpoint Your Comfort Food Triggers

Seek to write down what you eat and get a better understanding of how uncomfortable you are eating. "Maintaining a food journal for one week will help you assess the periods when you appreciate comfort or take responsive, healthier choices," Balk says. "When dinner is normally fried before major tests or meetings, comfort food, it is worth stopping the process and replacing the feeling with healthy options or getting comfort differently."

7. Get A Good Night's Sleep

Every nutritionist with whom we spoke mentioned the positive impact of adequate sleep at night on the levels of cortisol. Depending on our sleep cycles, Cortisol rises and falls: it is highest just after we wake up and lowest just before we reach the hay. It is also not surprising that sleep and cortisol levels are intertwined so heavily.

"Since cortisol levels are correlated with circadian rhythms, it will help keep cortisol levels stable for you to sleep at least 7-8hours each night," explains White. According to the researchers at Wake Forest, people who are sleeping for five or fewer hours have two-and-a-half times as much belly fat, while those that are sleeping for more than eight hours have only a little less.

8. Laugh It Off

Believe it or not, a good laugh will go a long way to decrease the levels of cortisol. "One way to reduce cortisol support for research is by deep, sincere laughter," says Steven M. Sultanoff, Ph.D. "Studies have shown that intense, sincere laughter for 10-20 minutes decreases serum cortisol.

White is in tune, saying that a positive mood will help get the job done: "Why you intend to improve your mood every day," he says. "It will raise cortisol levels and stress levels."

9. Break A Sweat

"The high-intensity exercise will induce cortisol development for around 15-20 minutes," says King. You need a particular type of exercise to decrease it. "To help reduce cortisol rates, aim to switch from extreme to moderate and low-intensity exercises such as strength training, yoga, pilates, and walking," she says.

According to a study in the Journal of Endocrinological Research, low-intensity exercise reduces the circulating level of cortisol.

10. But Don't Hit The Gym Too Often

The same study from the Journal of Endocrinological Studies found, by comparison, that low to high-intensity exercise contributes to a rise in cortisol levels circulating. In other words, more may not be better when it comes to exercise. A separate study in 2012 confirmed that long-term cortisol exposure in endurance athletes was significantly higher.

As a clinical psychologist, PsyD — a.k.a. PsyD. The weighing loss therapist says, "To skip the second trip to the fitness center and to take it easy can also be useful for reducing the levels of cortisol. [We have evidence] that over-exercise can increase the hormone.

11. Drink More Tea

There is a reason why people will relax by drinking tea. Research shows that tea reduces the level of cortisol. Besides, drinking about half a cup of green tea each day will reduce the risk of developing depression and dementia. Regular tea use was also linked to improved heart health. Just this year, a new study on tea and cardiac disease were published in the European Journal for Preventive Cardiology. The study showed that those who drank tea on average three times a week lived 1.5 years longer than those who did not drink it frequently or at all. Coronary heart disease.

12. Take A Walk Outside

Imagine that a doctor has given you a natural drug, or if you have been told to step outside for stress relief. How are you going to react? A study published in the newspaper from 2019, Frontiers in Public Health found that taking a 20-minute (minimum) walk in nature reduces cortisol levels significantly.

"Health care practitioners should use our results as evidence-based recommendations to prescribe a natural pill," said Dr. Mary Carol Hunter, University of Michigan Associate Professor and lead author of this investigation in the report, in a statement. "It provides the first assessments of how nature encounters stress levels in everyday life. This breaks new ground in resolving some of the problems of calculating an appropriate dose of nature."

13. Meditate

Perhaps one of the simplest and fastest ways to relieve stress is by meditation. In 2013, for instance, researchers at UC Davis published a study on meditation and cortisol levels in Health Psychology. What did they found? What did they found? This was correlated with lower levels of cortisol that the mind concentrated on what is happening at the moment rather than letting this wander through past and future experiences.

"The more people report their cognitive skills and their task immediately, the less cortisol they have to reside in," said Tonya Jacobs, a postdoctoral student at the UC Davis Center and writer of the study in a statement.

14. Do Yoga, Often

In many ways, yoga and meditation go hand in hand with positive health outcomes. A 2017 study in the journal Frontiers in Human Neuroscience found that daily meditation and yoga practice are due to lower levels of stress. Participants practiced meditation and yoga every day for three months. Following the retreat, participants reported improvements in "inflammatory signs," suggesting their tolerance to increases in stress levels. A further impressive result? Several participants also demonstrated improved depression and anxiety.

15. Eat More Cortisol-Lowering Foods

Believe it or not, certain foods can help reduce cortisol levels.

- dark chocolate

- bananas and pears

- probiotics in yogurt

For instance, a study published in the journal Antioxidants in 2019 examined the effects on cortisol levels of participants of dark chocolate consumption. The findings of the small study suggest that the average intake of just 25 grams of dark chocolate (think two squares of Intense Dark Ghiradelli, 86% cacao) is likely to minimize the total levels of cortisol.

HOW TO IMPROVE MOTIVATION

People like Bill Gates, founder of Microsoft, Sir Edmund Hillary of Mount Everest, and Maya Angelou may seem like a superhuman, but they're just like us. The only difference is that they stayed inspired until their goals were achieved. We all have goals, but it's easy to lose your drive. However, if you are persistent, you can achieve your dreams. In having the right mentality, you can boost your motivation. You can also change how you work towards your goals and overcome the delay.

A. Creating the Right Mindset

1. Choose A Mantra Or Set Of Mantras That Motivate You

You can create a slogan or use a quote yourself. Create your habit of saying your mantra aloud during the day at scheduled times, like getting up, lunch, or just before bedtime. Posting the mantras is also helpful.

- Good mantras include "every day is a new beginning and an opportunity for progress," "I am strong, powerful and able to accomplish my objectives," and "I can accomplish them if I think so."

- You can use simple notes like post-it notes to post your mantras, or you can use art prints with a quote. Put them in your refrigerator, in your mirror toilet, or on your house walls. Pick a place every day you see them.

2. Use Positive Self-Talk

Everybody has an internal voice, not always friendly. But turning that voice into the positive can improve your life. You can do this by catching and reframing negative thoughts positively. Besides, tell yourself about yourself, your future, and your goals consciously.

- Your mind can say to you, for example, "You 're not well enough." You may turn around and say, "I 'm good enough, but sometimes I get frustrated with the challenges. Things will look different tomorrow.

- In general, say things to yourself, "I am proud of myself for working hard every day," "I've done a lot, and the best thing is yet to come" and, "I know that I can do this if I continue to work hard."

3. Boost Your Confidence Via An Accomplishment

This is especially useful for people with long-term goals. Complete a mini target that is connected to your long-term objective or do something that's always daunting. Bear in mind that doing something can only mean trying.

- For instance, if you intend to play your music, you will increase your confidence by participating in an open mic night.

- If you feel you 're in a life rut, you can do something daring from the bucket list, like skydiving. This gives you a sense of control over what you do with your life, which helps to inspire you.

4. Reframe activities that you don't enjoy

It is normal not to enjoy your journey to your destination. You may love your work, but you hate parts of your workday, or you may want to have a cross country marathon, but hate hills. You can shift your vision by imagining it dimming and then incorporating new emotions. Imagine, for example, your stress on deadlines is gone, then imagine how good you feel when you complete a project.

- • Focus on the aspects you enjoy or benefit from these activities. For starters, it may be hard to walk hills, but it also provides you with a better view of the countryside.

- One way to do this is to concentrate on what you do and feel while you do not enjoy the activities. You may hate working meetings, for example, but concentrate on changing the landscape, talking with your fellow workers, or making a good impression on your boss.

5. Connect With Others Who Share Your Goals

Make friends on a journey like you, or join a group for like-minded people. They can be terrific motivators to keep track of it and can even be useful in times of difficulty.

- Look for like-minded friends in your destination online or in places. For example, to meet other aspiring musicians, you could attend an open mic night.

- You can also search for groups on meetup.com websites.

- Don't waste time with those who take you down. Choose the motivators instead.

6. Compare Yourself To Past You, Not Others

It is so tentative to compare yourself with others, but it is always an error. Regardless of how well you do, you always rank second. Connect yourself to you better! Remember where you have been in the past and now. Try to be better than you were before.

- When you catch yourself comparing yourself to others, remember that you will most probably see their highlight – not every day's nitty-gritty. You and yourself are the only rational contrast.

- Make a list of your positive features and achievements

to remember how far you have already gone!

7. Make A Gratitude List

By recognizing everything you must thank, you can create the positive attitude you need to remain motivated. Write down in your life all the good things, especially the things you have worked hard to get. Post your list somewhere you can see it, for example, on the fridge or lock screen of your telephone.

- It is best to make lists of gratitude often. You could even write down three to five items for which you are grateful every day.

- Over time, the appreciation list will make you feel better about life, helping to increase your drive to continue focusing on what is important to you.

B. Working Towards Goals

1. Keep your goals small and measurable.

It's cool to have big ambitions, but to make them easier to achieve; you have to will them. Break the bigger objectives into smaller ones. Then identify parameters for evaluating them.

- Your main aim, for example, will be to write a book. You might set yourself a small goal to construct a contour or complete a segment. This target is easy to calculate because the outline or chapter would be completed.

- Similarly, the major goal might be to run a marathon. You could set a small goal to run a 5K. You can calculate this aim by measuring how far you go every day or by registering for a race.

2. Create An Action Plan For Your Goals

You can build an ambitious strategy to meet your big objective, or you can limit it to your specific objectives. Include what you want to do, what you are going to do, and how you evaluate your success.

- For example, your big goal might be to run the marathon, and your small objectives could be to run a mile, 5K, 10K, and run a half marathon.

- Don't get stuck in the details. Write out a basic framework for your action plan and then work towards your objectives. You can modify or add to the scheme later.

- Keep brief with a short description. You don't have to prepare all the details. For example, you can start your marathon action plan by focusing on steps you must take to run a full mile, including purchasing new shoes, downloading a running app, and running three times a week.

3. Display Your Action Plan Where You Can See It Every Day

You can post it at home, place it in your calendar, or make it your digital wallpaper. See if you're on target every day. Often it's all right to get behind; however, your action plan will keep you on track.

- Seek to add your strategy to your fridge.

- Post your design there if you have a workspace.

- Choose a position that you can conveniently connect to.

4. Connect Hard Tasks And Obstacles Back To Their Purpose

It helps you get through and continue when things are hard. Each goal comes with hard work and challenges, and motivation to decrease is natural. You will remain inspired by giving more meaning to these tough times.

For example, it is not fun to run bleachers on your local track, but they will boost your physical fitness and help your athletic achievement.

Likewise, a lot of criticism of a poem that you wrote may discourage you, but it can help improve your poem and develop as a writer.

5. Track Your Progress

See how far you have come can be a great motivator! Keep track of all the milestones, large and small. Just one step towards your target is a success, so give credit to yourself!

- • Write down all your achievements so that when you feel discouraged, you can read about them.

- • You can even visually remember your development. • You could put up a poster with a trail on it if your target is to run a marathon. Divide the trail into 26.2 different parts. Whenever you increase your gap, color in a different segment.

6. Reward Yourself For Hard Work And Persistence

Rewards motivate you to keep up with your goal. Choose an enticing reward for you. Consider something that helps you to accomplish your goals, if possible. Here are some fantastic thoughts:

- You could be rewarded by sticking to the goal of writing a new notebook every day.

- Get a massage that will reward you for meeting your

goals.

- After turning off plans, enjoy a special meal with friends to help you achieve your goal.

- Treat yourself to a bubble bath.

- To celebrate your kickboxing success, buy a pair of weight gloves.

- Give yourself a yoga session.

- Take advantage of a good book.

7. Do Something You Enjoy Every Day

Just working towards something that you enjoy can be daunting, so take your time. Please spend at least a few minutes per day enjoying yourself, whether it is an episode of a favorite television show or a favorite treat or a friend's coffee. This helps you to stay motivated when times get rough.

8. Prepare Yourself For Setbacks

Setbacks are part of life, and all of them happen. They 're not saying you 're a loser! Create a quick outline of how you can conquer any challenges and know that you can.

- For instance, you may want to talk to a friend, take a day to brainstorm solutions, and then complete a small task to help you achieve your goal.

- Inform yourself, "Everything is part of the trip. As I have conquered them in the past, I will conquer this challenge.

C. Beating Procrastination

1. Spend Time Working On Your Goal Every Day

If you are working successfully towards your goal, the body releases dopamine, the hormone that makes you take action. Fortunately, with even a small amount of progress, you can increase your dopamine. Even if you can work only for 15 minutes on a certain day to reach your goal, you can see results.

2. Avoid Overthinking About Your Work And Goals

Too much thought can be detrimental for two reasons. First, it keeps you in your head and prevents you from acting. Furthermore, it allows you to worry about future issues that would possibly never happen. When you get lost in your thoughts, take action, begin with a small mission. You will be back on track when you check the mission.

When you begin to overthink, write down your thoughts, then try to draw up a to-do list so you can concentrate. You may not be able to deal with all your problems today, but some progress can be made.

3. Build Your Routines Around Your Goals

If you work on personal or professional goals, routines are important. Get used to setting aside time blocks to complete the activities you need to do.

For example, get up every day early to focus on your task, like going for an early morning run or working on your novel for an hour.

Every day, start your workday the same way. For example, you could review your to-do list for the easiest things that day, answer e-mail messages, or develop a regular action plan.

Develop a routine after lunch that helps you get on track again. For example, after lunch, you might arrange all your meetings to help you get back on track immediately.

4. Take Control Over Your Schedule

People and other activities can take part of your time. It's up to you to adjust your life and make sure you have time for it all. It means that you often have to say "no" to certain things to make room for others. Don't live your life as others like – spend your time doing what is important to you.

Plan meetings for you to achieve personal goals. You can also do things that make you content with this time.

5. Learn To Say "No" To Things You Don't Want To Do

It's all right to say no without guilt when someone asks for your time and conflicts with working towards your goal. Set your time limits and practice saying "no" to strangers. When the time comes, praise the individual and then turn it down gently.

Say, "It sounds so fun to your Halloween party, but that day I have already committed something."

You don't need to explain why, so don't feel pressured to justify your decision.

6. Ask For Help If You Need It

Sometimes you may be deterrent because you have had problems such as a hard task or lack of resources. Ask for help when this happens! Often someone wants support.

For example, you would need the person you live with to slack the house to meet a deadline.

You can ask your running friends to help you stay hydrated over long periods.

You can buy a piece of equipment you need.

OVERCOMING PSYCHOLOGICAL BLOCKS TO WEIGHT LOSS

There could be a psychological block in your way if you've tried any diet and exercise plan and can't slim down. Weight loss is a battle uphill for all, but emotional fights will take a longer time to reach their goals. The first step towards a safe solution is to recognize the problem. You may find there is more than one roadblock. The good news, however, is that these challenges can be resolved.

The Link Between Emotions and Weight Loss

Most of us have good intentions to eat better and exercise more often. And most of us know the essential things to eat and to stop. Yet we still end up derailing our progress when we feel tired, anxious, bored, or irritated even with our best intentions. And let's face it ... these feelings are often popping up.

We are just habituated creatures. Comfort is contained in routine. And, naturally, you search for such comfortable routines when you have trouble if your routine involves diet and activity patterns that have contributed to a bad weight. Such patterns relieve discomfort — at least in the short term.

What's worse, you probably have strong rational skills to sustain unhealthy habits. After all, why should you consider practicing relaxation and comfort? It is especially difficult to change our behaviors in the case of food behaviors. Our bodies are meant for eating. And when we do, we feel better. But not everything is lost if you want to change your weight loss habits. Weight loss counseling works somehow against you, but it does work for you with others. Before getting around the roadblock, you may need to find out what the roadblock is.

Common Psychological Blocks to Weight Loss and Maintenance

These are the most common emotional problems when people fight to slim down. Check the list to see if someone looks familiar.

All-or-Nothing Thinking

If you walk a fine line between completely sticking to your food plan or falling off the road, you might encounter a cognitive distortion called all or nothing, though. The term "cognitive distortion" is used by psychologists to mean persistently exaggerated thoughts that do not conform to what happens in the real world.

People who experience all or nothing when trying to lose weight think that their food choices are either a complete success or a total failure. Research has shown that a thought-style of something or nothing is closely related to a perceived lack of control over food and an inability to maintain a healthy weight. Some researchers have compared this lack of control to the actions of Jekyll and Hyde.

Unless you do not think so, you usually struggle with a little indulgence to return to a balanced eating schedule. Then, you would simply throw your towel and overeat because your diet fails absolutely.

Negative Body Image

If you try to change the size of your body and its shape, you may be less than satisfied with the current way it looks. Of course, there's nothing wrong with improving your health or appearance. But if your body image is too negative, the weight loss process can be impeded.

Researchers have demonstrated that in those who are obese, body dissatisfaction is more common than in those who are normal in weight. A negative corporal image is also associated with unhealthy eating patterns and other problems. For example, weight and shape concerns can also be embarrassed in the public domain, avoidance of self-consciousness, and excessive feelings of fatness after eating, say, study authors.

It is not clear whether a bad body image leads to unhealthy food or whether unhealthy food leads to a negative body image. What is clear is that a strong dissatisfaction with your body can prevent you from gaining a healthy weight.

Stress

There's a good reason for the name of comfort food. Most people feel good about eating. And some people use food as the best way to calm their emotions during times of stress. Although in people of all sizes and forms, this occasional strategy is not uncommon, it can create problems if you are trying to lose weight.

Studies have found that excessive consumption can become a chronic management mechanism for stressful lives. The strategy may be more common among the overweight.

And it's not just excessive food that can be problematic. Your food choices will probably change if you feel more anxious. Research published in Physiology and Behavior found that we eat more not only when depressed, but also that foods eaten are foods that are usually avoided for weight loss or reasons of health.

Depression

Studies are not sure whether depression induces weight gain or whether depression prevents loss of weight. Yet many scientists think there's a link. And even among people with average weight, depression can be troublesome in weight terms. Evidence has indicated that overweight perception raises psychological distress and can contribute to depression.

Symptoms associated with depression, such as sleeplessness or inactivity, may make weight loss harder. And some widely prescribed antidepressants can also contribute to weight gain.

Personal or Childhood Trauma

Several studies have found that people at higher risk of obesity are vulnerable to physical violence, sexual harassment, or peer bullying. Those with emotional trauma can change their eating habits to the degree that they affect their weight. Some scientists suggest that weight gain can be used for survivors of violence as an emotionally safe "solution."

Not everyone with personal or childhood traumas strives to keep their weight stable. Yet there may be a link if you have witnessed violence, neglect, or bullying.

Tips to Overcome Barriers

You might have found that you are familiar with one or more of the common psychological barriers to weight loss. It is not unusual to face multiple barriers on a healthy journey. However, these roadblocks do not have to prevent your success.

Each of the following tips and suggestions will overcome many obstacles. These suggestions are also healthy wellness strategies that have no side effects and are almost entirely free. Consider trying to find one or more of these solutions.

Keep a Journal

Stress avoidance is not always possible. However, you can identify and do your best to avoid certain situations or people that undermine your success. Maintaining a food journal can be helpful. Also, limited research has shown that maintaining a food journal can double the effects of weight loss.

Are you overeating or eating unhealthy food in certain environments or around certain people? Can you identify certain situations that make you feel uncontrolled and comfortable? A journal will help you assess these circumstances so you can restrict or fully prevent your exposure.

Make Small Changes

When something or nothing is thought that keeps you from adhering to your food schedule, consider taking small steps, and setting short-term goals.

Second, find a positive transition that is fair and achievable. You can want to walk every day for 15 minutes after dinner. Sets a goal for a week to focus on this goal. If you keep a food log, write down each day's information on various ways you have achieved in moving the goal forward.

Note, success is not your goal, but any effort to step in the right direction is progress, of which you must be proud.

Listen to Self-Talk

Watch out for the messages you send to yourself all day long? These recurrent thoughts can create a roadblock to good weight loss.

Many that are susceptible to a negative view of their body will find themselves hearing negative messages about their body every day. Phrases such as "I'm so fat" or "I'm so out of shape" spoken loudly or loudly in your head that weaken your ability to take a healthier move when the chance is there.

Listen to your inner conversation for a week or two. Identify a message or two that can encourage a negative self-image. Replace these messages with a mighty mantra. Phrases such as "my body are strong," "I 'm strong enough," or "I have come a long way" are widely used to build confidence.

Learn Relaxation Techniques

If you can not avoid difficult individuals or environments, relaxation strategies can be a safe alternative to emotional control in stressful situations.

Researchers have found that a particular kind of relaxation technique, known as guided imaging, can help with weight loss. You should work with a therapist to learn directed imagery, but guided imagery should be learned yourself. This takes time for you to learn, but controlled imaging can be the most powerful tool for weight loss in stressful times if your emotions cause you to feed.

Prioritize Sleep

Studies have consistently found that sleep patterns are related to stress, depression, and poor eating behaviors. So, to change your bedtime routines is one of the simplest, most calming moves to overcome psychological obstacles.

Consider your bedroom a sleeping sanctuary. Disable electronics (TV, monitor, cell phone) and do whatever you can to minimize noise. Get light-blocking sheets or buy a cost-effective sleep mask so that the night is completely dark. Many people are often raising the thermostat to facilitate restful sleep. Try to go to bed every night and wake up every morning at the same time.

Seek Help

Most professionals are specially qualified to deal with stress, past trauma, and other issues that may impede successful weight loss. A mental health professional can address the underlying emotional causes of alcohol eating and rise in weight.

Your doctor may be in a position to provide a referral. Other ways to find a therapist, if not. The American Psychological Association offers resources to help consumers find practitioners in your area, including a localizer.

If you do not see a behavioral health professional in your situations, suggest one of the recently created applications or technological platforms that include email, Skype, or facetime mental health consultation. These therapy services often provide relief for far less than personal advice.

COMMON WEIGHT-LOSS BARRIERS

Whether you have faced weight loss hurdles, you 're not alone. All have challenges unique to their particular journey to weight loss. You can become an obstacle to a safe loss of weight in the circumstances of your life, stress, income, time, biology and body photos, but this does not mean that you can not try to resolve them. Many people should face roadblocks to achieve their weight loss targets. Those who manage to lose weight and keep it off are those that learn to break their weight loss barriers as they arise. Here, we describe some common obstacles and practical tips to resolve them.

The Types of Weight Loss Barriers

You have to look through the first step to deal with your setbacks. You will develop some of the skills to rise above them once you know your obstacles. Know that many of the challenges you encounter were previously faced. It is not always easy to eat healthily and adhere to an exercise schedule. Most people have ups and downs along the way.

Many obstacles to weight loss are viewed as barriers, and the barrier is focused on your thoughts or feelings. Perceived obstacles may be as large and actual as concrete barriers, including barriers such as health conditions and physical restrictions. Whether your problems are perceived or specific, most can be further classified into three main categories: physical, emotional, and environmental.

1. Physical Barriers to Weight Loss
Popular physical obstacles are fatigue, pain, and underlying

medical conditions. Factors like fatigue and lack of sleep can also play a part in weight loss. While these challenges may be important, there are ways to conquer them and still lose weight.

Communicate With Your Physician

Talk to your doctor about your weight loss struggles. There may be a medical problem that contributes to your frustration.

For instance, weight gain may be caused by certain medicines (including steroids, birth control pills, and some depression medications). You may experience weight gain if you have recently stopped smoking. Hormonal changes (such as those in menopause) can increase weight loss and lead to weight gain. And weight gain is associated with medical conditions, including PCOS and other thyroid disorders.

Expand Your Healthcare Team

Ask your doctor for references to a registered dietitian, physical therapist, psychologist, and/or obesity specialist. These experts will customize your recovery plan to help your objectives. For a doctor's recommendation, there is typically a greater likelihood that insurance benefits are provided. Check your contract to see what your coverage is going to cover. Speak to the specialist office to inquire if necessary about out-of-pocket prices.

Improve Your Sleep

Researchers found that not sleeping enough would disrupt your metabolism. Researchers have shown that your hormonal balance will change if you don't get the requisite sleep and have increased hunger and appetite. Indeed, evidence shows that people who get less than seven hours of sleep are more likely to be obese or overweight.

The good news is that changing your sleep routine can help you slim down. Experts suggest sleeping, sleeping in a cool dark room at the same time, and eliminating electronic devices (like tablets and mobile phones) to promote a calming atmosphere.

Get Hydrated

Simple changes to your everyday routine will encourage weight loss. Staying hydrated is an easy change that has many health benefits and can even help you slim down. Studies have also shown that drinking more water is related to better weight loss outcomes.

The feelings of hunger and thirst are not uncommon. Keep your refrigerator packed with water bottles to grab and go. If you want, add berries or other ingredients (e.g., basil or cucumber). When you are eating in the kitchen all day, try drinking several ounces of water before you eat to see if this satisfies your appetite.

Do Your Homework

Research various exercise plans and healthy cooking tips. Habits leading to weight loss can be managed when it's fun. For example, if you are faced with obesity, pain, or joint issues, non-weight bearing exercises such as water aerobics can be relaxing. Make improvements to your daily meal schedule by enrolling in an interactive cooking class where you can learn new ways to prepare meals or vegetables and have fun in the kitchen.

2. Environmental Barriers to Weight Loss

Some of the reasons you find it difficult to lose weight may be about your environment. If you don't endorse a balanced diet and practice program in your setting, you may feel like you are fighting a losing battle. Weight loss at times can seem impossible by environmental restrictions, including restricted access to nutritious food or exercise facilities, inadequate social support, or lack of time due to financial, family, and professional pressures.

Talk to the People Around You

Get family and friends help by expressing your needs. Be specific about how you can help your plan succeed. That your wife can take on extra duties or your children can help more in the home. Your staff may be prepared to support your healthy lifestyle by providing wellness or flexibility in your work schedule. A successful work is an efficient worker (most of the time). Thankfully, more and more businesses have started to understand the benefits of health programs.

Get Creative With Exercise

If you are going to the gym, there are plenty of home training options available. Rent or buy DVDs, search the Fitness plan for your TV schedule, or find free workouts online. There are also plenty of smartphone and tablet apps for workouts. You will find various classes and tips, forums, and other resources.

You can also use the resources outside your doorstep to get in shape. Walking is a great way to practice. Drive along the local trails, go up the stairs of your office or apartment complex, or schedule a weekend family stroll. Many shopping malls offer walkers special hours to practice before the crowds take over.

3. Emotional Barriers to Weight Loss

It seems counterintuitive to say you want to lose weight, but your thoughts about losing weight deter you. Nevertheless, emotional weight loss barriers are well known and often relevant. These obstacles can include skepticism about your ability to achieve your goals, negative associations, high levels of stress, or simply lack of motivation.

Enlist the Help of a Qualified Professional

Many mental health professionals (including social workers, therapists, and psychologists) concentrate on body weight emotions. If your weight issues have already been discussed for potential medical purposes, consider talking to a therapist about emotional problems.

Learn to Motivate Yourself

Motivation is a learning skill. Techniques such as constructive self-talking and journalistic are also established ways to improve your confidence and to push you in the right direction. Self-monitoring has also proven to be an important method for losing weight. Self-surveillance may involve maintaining a food diary, daily weigh-ins, or monitoring your physical activity using a paper log, fitness tracker, or app. The self-monitoring method lets you track your everyday actions to raise consciousness so that improvements can be made if necessary.

Use Stress-Reduction Techniques

Stress-related to your busy life, family issues, lack of success in weight loss, or an underlying health condition can lead easily to emotional eating and weight gain. Also, the development of obesity was associated with chronic stress.

On the other hand, weight loss effects have been shown by stress management strategies (such as deep breathing or guided visualization). You can learn methods of stress reduction, such as breathing, meditation, or journaling. Plan these things into your day to remain in the right mood for success.

POWERFUL PRACTICES FOR RELEASING EMOTIONAL BAGGAGE, HURT AND REGRET: LETTING GO OF THE PAST TO LIVE A BETTER LIFE

Releasing Emotional Baggage: It's Time to Let Go of the Past

To build a solid base that encourages your advancement toward a Well Life, you should do all kinds of things to improve yourself. However, how you simultaneously weaken this base will thwart all the fortification of the world. You can only go so far as to avoid unresolved disputes, forgive and exclude religions from your history. And you must be very honest and learn to let go of your baggage to achieve Well Life.

Do you have broken deals, unstable marriages, rebellions, or minimal stories? It can be an uncomfortable process to clean up this conflict by letting go of the past, but you probably already suffer from some uncomfortable situation because these issues have not been addressed or solved.

What's Wrong with Keeping the Past in the Past?

Now, we would like to tell you before you say, "Oh boy, it's going to be hard," that leaving the past must not be a difficult experience. In reality, letting go is a chance to feel lighter. It's just that there's often something between weight and lightness, which one of our former teachers called a "vigil of discomfort." The discomfort is a shield because it is quite insubstantial. As soon as we can feel it, we pass it easily. And lightness and potential are on the other hand!

Let's explore how these loose ends of the past can affect you and how necessary it is to let go of rage and other negative emotions. One thing that could happen when you are ready for something exciting (whether it's a new relationship, a career change or a cross-country move) is that your subconscious quickly gets through all of your baggage – unresolved issues, past traumas, failures, losses – and decides that this is a bad idea.

Instead of hating your mind, it is important to remember that you have this mind trained. You began as a baby with a clean mind, and you gradually trained your mind to look for things that might put your survival or happiness in jeopardy. Your mind is designed to function like that. It happens that most people are too willing to do this job. The more the negative memories of your life are compounded, the deeper they 're in your mental memory, and the more important it is to take the life seriously.

The mind looks for something in the present, which even remotely resembles past experiences to help you avoid repeating them. This produces alert thought and initiates intense emotions to grab your attention.

So what can you do to let go and move forward? Thank you for your efforts to protect you, but remind you that your views and generic data are outdated. This is a great step to let the past go. There is no point in blaming yourself for the way your mind works. You have done your best with the tools at your fingertips at any moment. But if you want freedom, without being limited by your background, to show up to any moment, it is necessary to realize that your baggage prevents this. The restricting beliefs and reminders of past feelings are an intrusion into your room and the harmony inside.

Learning to Let Go: Figure Out What's Holding You Back

The key to identifying and letting go of past incidents that are prioritized cleanups is that you do not feel light or clean when you bring them to mind and then inspect your body. You may feel heavy, tight, restless, or restricted instead. Or negative emotions like guilt, fear, shame, anger, regret, sadness, or grief might come up.

You may not be able to give an especially strong physical or emotional answer to something you did that was objectively bad. In such cases, it is important to remember that an event 's goal of "sin rating" is smaller than a hook. On the other hand, as you think about it, you may have mistakenly thrown away your children's first finger painting and felt an overwhelming sense of remorse.

Create a table to let go of the past and release the luggage you hold back. Write "My Baggage List" at the top of a piece of paper and build five separate columns on your piece with the following headers: problem, fault, result, chance, fix.

Column 1: What Are Your Issues?

Write three unresolved situations in this column. These could be stuff that happened in the past that you haven't let go of (maybe you had your time talking in white pants in your school).

- Problems that occur right now (you may be overweight and hate, or in an on-going argument with your boss)

- Issues involving other people (You ran across the hairless cat of Mrs. McGillicuddy)

- Situations that are thoroughly lived (You stole a candy bar from the convenience store)

If you have difficulties thinking of things while you are learning to let go, try and ask yourself: What do I dislike or deplore about myself, my life, others, or the world? And, who (from my own life) would I least like to be trapped in a lift? Then search for unresolved issues through your responses. Letting others go starts by knowing how you are being held, hostage. At this point, however, do not seek to go through your entire life. Only start with the first few things you can think of. You don't need to explain the entire situation in the issue column when you decide which issues you are working on as part of the letting go of the past; just use a few keywords ("candy bar"), to help your mind connect with it.

Column 2: Who Are You Blaming?

It's now time to decide who you blame for each of your problems. What are you kept in your head as a hostage? What do you hold forgiveness from? In this column, write their name or names. The answer here is possible (and common) to be me.

The Power of Forgiveness

Consider letting your past rebellions go as a mental purification before you begin to restore your new life. There is so much discussion in the world of natural health about how our bodies can be cleansed, but so little about how to cleanse our minds. Forgiveness is the most effective tool for emotional cleaning.

Recognize that most people are just children who are confused (or at least we can be emotional).

We are still looking to meet our needs, still wanting the approval of everyone, So when we're upset, we often work from a perspective that's not very different from when we were six years old. Learning to let go requires understanding this viewpoint and embodying empathy.

During our lifetime stumbling, we also cause pain to others. If you are on the receiving end, it might be important to consider that they were confused: they didn't understand that they would meet their needs without hurting someone else, they didn't understand the impact of their actions, they didn't know the love they always had, and they didn't understand the nature of their connection. This might not be all right for you, but hopefully, it is an opportunity for forgiveness. With this understanding, it is much easier to let go of the frustration and shift from the past.

Consider the possibility that lifelong punishment may be unreasonable.

If it is your intención to withhold forgiveness of someone (possibly yourself) for the rest of your lives, then this is defined as "cruel and unusual." Ask yourself: How long will I wait until it's enough? Or how long will I pollute myself with this?

View forgiveness as something we do for ourselves as much as for the other person.

When you fail to forgive others, you ultimately take on the responsibility of imposing a punishment instead of forgiving the past. Yeah, in the mental prison, you play the warden, and it takes energy and emotional "bandwidth." Are you going to give the very person you think you have wronged his freedom and your peace of mind? Will it, in some way, change the situation by corrupting your happiness and restricting your inner freedom?

Resentment is the system's mental poison. Even if you want to do nothing nice for the person you've been resenting, you have to get this poison out for your own sake by letting this anger go. The good part is that you are relaxed instantly. You can quit the gardening job and detox the poison in the same act.

See forgiveness not as a single act, but as an ongoing commitment.

It may often not be possible for you just to pronounce someone forgiven, and that is the end. As we said, strong feelings cut deep grooves; falling into them is easy. Instead, you may need to commit that from now on, you will recognize once you start to harbor resentment. And once you remember that you picked it up again, you can let it go again. Leaving the past is a process, and learning to let go takes practical action. You won't analyze why you have collected it again; you won't scold yourself that you have picked it up again, and you won't indulge in the resentment again. You are just going to lower it as quickly as possible (forgive them again). And you'll feel better almost. Soon, the habit of dropping it starts replacing the habit of keeping it.

This opponent part of you believes that someone has done something bad to you (and possibly others). Anything was not to have occurred that did happen. And at the same time, you and your current point of view are right. Maybe you build your case in the shower and driving.

The thing is, you block your progress in life and let go of the past when you are stuck in needing to be true. By holding on to it, you decrease your perspective. You do not see the big picture of what will most effectively bring you to a happy and fulfilling life.

Remember: the person who needs the most forgiveness is you.

If you are like almost all other human beings, to some extent, you blame yourself for everything in your life that you believe should be different, and that makes it difficult to let go of the past. You do not know, and you might blame someone else as well, but it is likely that when things are not good, your subconscious has an excuse that is similar to something is wrong with me, or maybe my body is wrong, my subconscious is wrong, I make wrong decisions, I have messed up my life, etc.

A self-limiting belief is like sandbags that weigh your hot air balloon. And if you forgive how to let go, it's like cutting the cords. When you begin to forgive yourself habitually, you not only begin to feel a lightness and freedom that is absent for many of us for decades, but you begin to realize how powerful you are. While it takes effort to let go and move on, it has advantages!

Column 3: Consequence

It is time to return to your lists of bags. Given the complaint in the first column, the person or persons that you blame and withhold forgiveness from the second column and the previous discussion, in the third column, what is the result of allowing this to remain unresolved? Even if you can't think of objective consequences that don't let anyone or a previous occurrence go, your peace of mind and space always carry the toll. For instance, if you argue with the boss unresolved, perhaps this causes you to fear the work you normally enjoy.

Column 4: Opportunity

How if you could just stop fighting and be at peace? What if you let go of the past problem? More happiness? More happiness? More energy? More energy? Freedom? Freedom? The desire to keep your life going?
Pen down your answer.

Column 5: Fix

This column demonstrates how you can solve this problem to free yourself to create your good Life. What action are you going to take to fix this problem? A determination to let it go if it occurs? A communication to resolve? A show of your confidence? A ritual of letting go of the past in which you or someone else release you from prison?

Here are some more suggestions to let someone go and move on:

If you have broken a contract, violated someone's trust, behaved with no honesty or other harm (and you may have been the recipient of that damage), accept what you have done, make no excuses and clean up. Do something that reflects the sincerity of your apology, to let go of the past. Go further — especially if your goal is to regain someone's (or your own) trust. Show 110 percent (or yourself) for them. Replace, fix, or refund what was stolen.

Often it is dangerous to confess a past mistake or to publicly repair an old wound to clean out your side of things. Do not if the other party has moved on or if it is not healthy or efficient to include them in your decision. Although we want you to heal your wounds, this is not always feasible or appropriate to let go of the past. In these instances, our concern is your healing, your forgiveness, restoring your confidence, and putting it behind you. To accomplish this, you can find besides a pledge to forgiveness an anonymous act of kindness, a donation to a charity, or a ceremony by yourself, for instance, planting a tree to symbolize new hope and good growth. Learning to let go often involves concentrating more on yourself than anybody else.

Most of the past transgressions which weighed on us included ways in which we didn't honor or hurt ourselves. In addition to forgiveness, we encourage you to show love for yourself actively. How can you demonstrate how much you love today? What nice stuff you could do for yourself? Why do you listen to yourself? How can you honor yourself more fully? This is not only an excellent exercise but a powerful method to let go of the past.

Consider abandoning the past by Dr. Ihaleakala Hew Len's forgiveness practice based on the old Hawaiian art of reconciliation, known as ho'oponopono. See yourself and repeat these four sentences, as if you were listening to yourself from your soul: "I love you. I'm so sorry. I'm so sorry. Forgive me, please. Thank you. "The use of these words as a mantra will help you get out of your prison and keep you safe. It can also be used by others.

It takes commitment and a willingness to be vulnerable to recovery and to let go of your past. Whenever you solve one of those problems, it's like dropping a case full of rocks. As you experience increasing freedom and lightness and continue to learn to let go, you will begin to identify and resolve conflicts and grievances, because your mind becomes aware of their weight. Your plans will be more successful at a clean beginning.

POSITIVE AFFIRMATIONS FOR WEIGHT LOSE

Permanent weight loss or weight control requires lifestyle changes. The statements given here will help you to change your lifestyle slowly but gradually. Use the optimistic affirmations below intelligently and consistently for weight loss. Weight loss or weight management is typically a clear feature of our lifestyle.

In other words, the meal we consume, the duration of the diet, the way we cook, the physical activity we endure, the rest we do, the mental mindset we hold for a long time-actually, throughout our entire lives-defines our weight and/or weight problems. Using an acceptable weight loss statement below to help with your question.

Most diets just work as long as the diet works! The moment diet stops, all the weight lost slowly begins to return. That simply means that you will have weight issues again if you don't change your lifestyle. Strong weight loss affirmations will help you in improving your lifestyle. The body has been found to maintain the weight with which the mind is relaxed. If the mind finds this necessary for some reason, the body starts to accumulate weight and very quickly becomes overweight.

For example, if it is beneficial during childhood to be a "big body" for security purposes, your subconscious mind would take it upon itself to make you big and then to maintain your health. It is impossible to lose the weight gained in this manner if the mind is not tackled first.

In such cases, no diet will ever help. It is necessary to change our thinking for real weight loss. With the new weight you want, you need to make your mind comfortable. Affirmations of weight loss will support you in this mission.

Obesity is sometimes due to glandular malfunction. Diets or affirmations will not work in such cases. You must receive the same medical treatment. If you are overweight, consult your doctor before starting a diet or affirmations on any problems with the gland.

Take care of the wording of the statement. Never say "I am not fat" because you concentrate on your question in this situation, that is, being fat. And whatever you concentrate on, develops. Concentrate on the solution. So say 'I'm slim' or 'I'm getting slimmer and slimmer every day.'

If you are a certain person, repeating over and over the following sentences, at least a hundred times a day, ideally before a mirror, for at least six months is sure to gradually but steadily make you look at and lead a different life, one more fit than fatter. As always, combine two or three of the free weight-loss claims or even write your safe weight-loss claims with the following phrases.

The 10 Affirmations

So, these are some of the best ten statements I've ever come to ... or made, actually wrote. And they will motivate you to shift your belief system tremendously.

1. I Am Healthy and Lean

The first is your body's confidence. "I want to be healthy and lean," you are in the space. I want to. Now that you say, "I'm healthy and lean," your body takes up the energy of that. When you claim it and the field of thought and celebrate it emotionally by feeling good about this truth, that is your real energy. If it weren't true, where you were would be perfectly happy. Your current state tells me that you are unhappy. This is true. Because you want the truth now to materialize so that you can claim the truth as if it is now, because when you create it. I'm healthy and lean. I'm healthy and lean. Make your self-identity the foundation. That's what your body wants to own. It is capable of building a healthy, lean state. It wants to be strong and lean. Believe in your body. Believe in your body.

2. I Give Myself Recognition Beyond Food

I recognize myself beyond food. How often are you treating yourself and using food as a reward? Yeah, I feel guilt too. I feel guilty too. Even the other day caught me, "Oh, I'm so, you know, I'm very excited. I've finished that. I'll go and eat something special. "I believe this links with our condition as kids because food has been used extensively to try and invoke cooperative behavior. "You are recompensed. Let me reward you here." As a parent, it's very difficult not to use food as a reward. "You could have a snack, yes. Only if ... "We continue with that pattern, and we use food as a way of self-recognition. That's what it's all about since we eat unhealthy foods more often because we prefer sweet therapies that are genuinely good when we use food for recognition.

3. I Love My Body

And, you'll go beyond that. I recognize myself beyond food. I love my body, and fat is just gone. Let yourself speak. Let yourself communicate. Are you conscious that your body is listening to you? Are you disgusted? Are you even saying that you hate your body? Look in the mirror and put it down, would you tell a close friend you love and appreciate what you say to your body? Your body listens to you. You listen. You listen to your fat cells. You 're going. You 're going. "Well, I suppose I'll answer that." Learn to love your body now.

We have this odd thing in our experience if we choose to love and embrace our body in a state we don't like, and we think we want to have it, such as, "Oh, I'm not careful. I'm apathetic, and now I'll always enjoy my body. It's never changing; I don't know. "No! Love is the highest vibration to bring about change. Whether you feel cherished, your body is inspired to improve. If your body has guilt and a shameful force, it wants to go over. This is not helped in good decisions. It's not going to feel like exercise. Love is going to push you into transition. I love my body, and fat is just gone.

4. I Am My Ideal Weight

Catch yourself, then. Look in the mirror, go, "What do you know? That's how it is. Right now, I'm going to love it. "I 'm going to use love as a tool for promoting progress in my body. Oh, sure, if you're in space, you 're going to put in, "No, that's not real." You have to build with a conviction what you want first. Believe it; you 're going to see it soon.

5. I Feel Great In My Clothes

In my shoes, I feel fantastic. It is challenging, as it's also difficult to feel amazing when you're not the size you don't want to be in the position that you do. I have a great system to support you. Seek my Dressing Your Truth link and go to caroltuttle.com. Right now, today, I can make you feel amazing in your clothes, no matter the size or shape. You want to look amazing in your clothes and declare them to be real and feel wonderful in my clothes. You 're going to build that.

6. I Am Saying No To Foods That Are Not Healthy For Me

How many things do you say yes to a trend you don't feel healthy? Even if you were collected to say no easily? Say no easily to foods you 're not healthy. This confidence will inspire you to choose. Avoid pouring money into poor food options and then build up arguments.

7. I Am Attracted To Foods & Resources Supportive For My Body

And here we have a kind of duality. I say no to this, and I'm drawn vigorously to this now. Like ... it feels like ... I feel moved. I feel engaged with it instantly. It's easy, not, "Oh, I've got to eat this. I 'm tired. I'm tired. You want to feel supported; you're attracted to it. I don't want to have to do this. I 'm drawn to the food and energy my body gets. I'm filled with statements that block my body 's pain.

8. I Am Full & Satisfied With The Proper Amount Of Food

I love this one. I love this one. How much less are you going to eat if the conviction goes on? I had enough. I wanted plenty. My appetite is full. I 'm done. I 'm done. I feel satisfied. I feel satisfied.

9. I No Longer Need The Extra Weight To Protect Me

All right. Good. It's becoming dangerous. Like, "Whoa, whoa, whoa, that's getting a bit of heavy-duty." Have you got some things that will help you with that one and just say that it's the truth because, "Whoa, whoa, you know, for some reason, I need the world 's security." Ok, I have some other resources that will help you fix this. And, you know, as a safety barrier, you don't need weight.

10. I Look In The Mirror & See A Healthy And Fit Body That I Love

And here, as you start practicing this at once, I see a healthy fit body I love in the mirror. Can you visualize the body you want to manifest? The body that wants to live? What body would you like to show yourself? Can you look in the mirror and see the potential there through your current experience? Use this trick. Use this trick. See it. See it. How are you supposed to look like? How are your legs going to look? Your arms, your torso? What are you going to feel about that? Act now as if it's happening. Show your appreciation and don't wait to get it from others.

Train Your Mind

Let's repeat all of them in a row, then. You can go back to that point of the video any time, particularly when you feel a craving, feel destructive, and sabotage yourself; I'll say it, repeat it. You feel discouraged. You feel discouraged. Just go through it. Pick three with which you truly, truly resonate. Three of your picks. Own Them. Own Them. Memorize them. Memorize them. Use them daily. You want to practice this to train your mind so that you can become your true system of belief, both your unconscious and your conscious mind. This is correct. For you, it's true. You insert it into your mind.

Let's go through them. Let's go through them. I'm sound and lean. After me, say it loudly. I recognize myself beyond food. I love my body, and fat is just gone. I am my optimum weight. I am my perfect weight. In my shoes, I feel fantastic. I say no to food that isn't safe for me. I am drawn to the food and energy that my body supports. I am pleased with the right quantity of food. I don't need additional weight to protect me anymore. I see a safe and balanced body I enjoy when I look in the mirror.

Other Weight Loss Affirmations to use daily

Weight loss can look like an uphill battle, and weight loss claims can make it easier for you to do so. Let's take a look at this huge list to help you on your journey to weight loss.

- The loss of weight naturally comes to me.
- I 'm happy to achieve my goals for weight loss.
- Every day, I lose weight.
- I love exercising regularly.
- I eat foods that help my health and well-being.
- I only eat when I'm starving.

- I see myself clearly at my ideal weight now.
- I love good food tastes.
- How much I eat, I'm in control.
- I love to exercise; it just makes me feel good.
- I get fitter and stronger by exercising every day.
- I'm easy to reach and keep my ideal weight
- I love my body and care about it.
- I deserve a lean, fit, attractive body.
- I'm constantly developing healthier eating habits.
- Each day I get slimmer.
- I look and feel fantastic. I look and feel amazing.
- To be healthy, I do what it takes.
- I 'm glad I've been redefining success.
- I choose to practice.
- Foods that make me look and feel good. I want to eat.
- I'm in charge of my health.
- I love my body. I love my body.
- I'm careful with making my body stronger.
- I exercise happily every morning when I wake up to maintain the weight loss I like.
- In shifting my eating habits from unhealthy to good, I stick to my weight loss plan.
- I 'm happy with every piece I make to lose weight in my big effort.
- I get slimmer and healthier every day.
- I 'm creating an enticing organism.
- I am cultivating a lively fitness lifestyle.
- I'm building and loving a body.
- Strong affirmations for weight loss
- Changes in my lifestyle change my body.

- I feel great now that in four weeks, I have lost more than ten pounds and can not wait until I meet my lady friend.
- I've got a flat belly.
- I admire my strength in making food decisions.
- I weigh 20 pounds less happily.
- I enjoy walking three to four days a week and do toning exercises at least three times a week.
- Eight glasses of water I drink a day.
- Every day, I eat fruit and vegetables and eat chicken and fish mostly.
- I learn and use positive intellectual, emotional, and spiritual skills. I'm ready to change!
- I 'm prepared to construct new thoughts about myself and my body.
- I love my body and respect it.
- It's exciting to discover my unique weight loss food and exercise system.
- I am the success story of weight loss.
- I 'm happy to be the right weight for me.
- I can easily adopt a balanced food schedule.
- I prefer to have trust thoughts about my ability to improve my life positively.
- It feels like shifting my body. Exercise is fun! Exercise is fun!
- I use deep breathing to assist me with tension and relaxation.
- I'm a lovely guy.
- I enjoy being at my ideal weight.
- I'm a delightful person. I want to love it. I deserve love. I may lose weight safely.

- I'm a good lower weight influence in the world.
- I remove my body's urge to attack.
- I accept my sexuality and enjoy it. It's all right to feel sensual.
- My metabolism is very good.
- I maintain the optimal health of my body.

These confirmations of weight loss will inspire you to lose weight.

Affirmations for Confidence

- I'm a trustworthy person who is respected everywhere.
- I am a unique and dignified person, and I deserve the respect of everybody.
- I accept myself, and for who I am, I love myself.
- What other people say matters little. What I respond to and what I believe in really matters to me.
- My mind is full of positive thoughts, and I understand and let go of negative patterns of thought.
- I breathe in relaxation and stress.
- And so do others around me, I respect myself.
- I'm happy with my life, and I choose to accept myself exactly as I am.
- All I have in my life, I love, and I live in utter happiness.
- I feel optimistic about the challenges of life, and I embrace them with joy, without guilt or fear.
- I substitute "I must," "I must," and "I must" with "I must."

- I trust myself and believe that I'm a worthy person who loves others.
- It's easy to meet new people. I can create supportive relationships without feeling anxious and make new friends.
- I consider my strengths and shortcomings, and I am actively working to change.
- I am a focused person, and when I feel challenged or wrong, I won't stop doing anything.
- I'm generous, caring, compassionate, and I look after the people around me.
- I inhale trust and exhale fear and anxiety.
- I'm a trustworthy person, and I always do exactly what I say. I have integrity. All of us can trust me.
- I have confidence and confidence in myself, and I have let the negative go.
- Being alive makes me glad.
- It is good and rewarding to be myself, and I always see challenges as opportunities to demonstrate my abilities.
- All that's good in this world, I deserve. I release every need for suffering, and I feel happiness, trust, and love entering my body, mind, and soul.
- I am enthusiastic and vigorous, and trust is an integral part of my nature.
- I'm healthy, well-cared, and beautiful, and I recognize my interior and outer beauty.
- I thrive on my absolute trust. My life is lovely, and I enjoy it every moment.
- As I understand my uniqueness, I never compare myself to others.

- As I inhale, confidence fills my entire being, and every time I exhale, all guilt and shyness are washed away.
- I embrace myself as I am, and with everything I do, I get stronger and better.
- I'm a guy who takes on new challenges easily.
- Change is inevitable, and I completely embrace it.

EXTREME WEIGHT LOSS HYPNOSIS: MYTHS ABOUT RAPID WEIGHT LOSS AND FAST DIETING (EXPERIENCE)

Many things sabotage people from proper, fast weight loss. Not only have people have their minds and anxieties to stop (which is why I help with hypnosis, NLP, and EFT), but myths also make people think incorrectly about fast, safe diets. How often have you heard "That's insecure about losing about 1 to 2 pounds a week." or "You never should skip your breakfast! It's just your metabolism!" or "Look how those French people eat! It's a minute! That's not enough!" "This can make your weight loss better by medicines and supplements!"

Okay, as a doctor, I, too, have learned these things from nutritionists, dieticians, and other doctors and specialists who still work in an old paradigm of the right and wrong diets. I'm here to share a new paradigm for breaking these myths so you can quickly and safely lose weight just like the body is meant to do.

As a doctor who helped 50 patients lose a total of 2000 pounds in five months or an average of 40 pounds in each, I can tell you that these myths are only impeded by healthy, safe, and rapid weight loss. And no! And no! These patients had NO gastric bypasses or lap ribbons! They used the natural weight loss tactics of their bodies to succeed.

Let's think about the mechanics of the body. We 're eating to remain alive. It gets fat when we eat extra. When we're not eating enough to support ourselves, the fat is burned to use what we have stored. It's that easy. This is the power of all mammals. Fat helps our body to hold sugar and nutrients alive and to vanish if we do not have enough to go into our mouths.

All these little variations to this simplicity, though, are used to confuse you and lead to the perpetuation of these myths.

1. "Losing more than 1-2 pounds a week is unsafe."

I guided my patients safely through low-calorie diets for 1 pound per day. It works, and it's healthy and how we've been programmed to use fat genetically. Often I think that people who use the first fallacy justify remaining on their diets or longer regimes. It sells gym memberships and sells monthly programs costing $50-1000 a month. If it's normal to lose only 1 pound a week, you can keep a person 80 pounds for 80 weeks on a diet! This is a great deal of cash! If you look at key health websites, there are many articles about losing more than 1-2 pounds a week, but you will find that they address fast, doctors-assisted weight loss for the poorest patients. Why do we, but not healthy patients, do it for them? I didn't distinguish, and the results were great. But yes, the patients lose weight under the supervision of a doctor, and I can make sure no weight loss issues.

With my weight loss programs, which I have given my patients, they lose 30 pounds over 30 days, 80 pounds over 80 days, 150 pounds over 150 days, etc. Today I had a patient who had lost 50 pounds in 50 days, who had taken three blood pressure medicines, who looks and felt great. Her blood pressure is 100/80 now when we started 150/90. Will it be easier for her to tell me a gradual weight loss so that she could have high blood pressure a day longer? I don't think so. I don't think so. In a quick amount of time, she is healthier and safer with my hypnosis and quick weight loss techniques.

2. "Don't skip breakfast. It's unhealthy in a diet, and you won't lose as much weight!"

Eating breakfast keeps the metabolism in line so that more calories are consumed all day long. This is true if you are constantly in weight. But when it comes to weight loss, eating breakfast is not a weight-loss accelerator. Calories still have to go somewhere. Yes, in the long run, you get more obese when you skip breakfast and then eat normal food for lunch and dinner afterward. An individual skips breakfast puts their body in the state of hunger so that any extra food you consume later in the day becomes fat as the body scraps to hold more sugar in the body after it is said to be hungry as breakfast is skipped.

However, if you miss breakfast to consume limited amounts of food for lunch and dinner (lower calorie amounts than a full day is necessary), your energy will be consumed by BURN FAT. So breakfast will burn excess fat in a lower calorie intake time. This is God's way of designing us. When we were hunter-gatherers and roamed the earth as nomads for the next food supply, sometimes winter would come, and food would drop, or there would be famine times when there were just no food supplies. During these times of food need, God was clever enough to design us with a sugar source. Both mammals have the so-called fat food storage system. If you see advertisements seeking assistance to children who are hungry in other countries, these children rely on these fat shops to survive the absence of ample nutrients.

God and nature built us to use this fat store HEALTHILY if we do not have ample food. We 're fasting, so anybody who tells you that weight loss is unhealthy by fasting argues with the Big Guy, who designed this survival system. Throughout time, the human body has adapted to the use of fat to store food to survive hunger or famine. If it were bad, it wouldn't work because evolution and nature were. The fittest survive, and fat storage systems survive longer if no food is available.

Here's how this system has been bastardized. After we passed the ice age and became agricultural in our economy, food supplies were abundant. We have no longer starving, and we no longer hunger because we have plenty of farms and food surplus to provide us with food right now. The supermarkets were bigger and larger, as our quick food is readily available. It's funny that we call quick food because while it is quick because of the fast service, it is the very food that keeps us from fasting. After all, it is readily available. We simply overindulge and never hunger, which leaves us with big food stores through obesity in our bodies.

Besides, in the last 15 years, we have added large amounts of sugar to our food as fillers and as fat replacements to enhance the flavor. So, in the middle-class Western hemisphere, we are no longer hungry, we give ourselves more calories than we need and are now more obese than ever before. (Don't get me started with our first-ever outbreak of obese 6-month-olds due to recent fructose add-ons).

So we're no longer hungry, but every time we go into a store, we get plenty of harvests. We have no chance of using our normal human system for storing and releasing sugar because people don't hunger, fat burning from the lack of calories.

It is where Gastric bypass, mouth plumbing, the techniques for lap belt come in. Instead of hunger, or food shortages or winters to naturally cause us to lose weight as expected, we use artificial operations to compel our most ill-healthy people, the chronically obese, to lose weight as Nature had intended. Required caloric droughts by surgery practice, however, for those overweight patients have high surgical risks. Through my own and colleagues' observations, I saw our patients die after sepsis procedures: cardiac attacks, surgical complications and anesthesia, undernourishment, iron deficiency anemia, vitamin deficiency, and suicide caused by depression. After the treatment, I have had one patient die from bulimia. Not everyone gets the psychological support they need, nor do they receive guidance as soon as they lose weight.

There was also a phenomenon of discontent and poor satisfaction with the results after losing weight. I speak of life fulfillment when I say happiness. Most people lose weight just to discover that the tremendous changes they were told would not exist in their lives. Guys who have lost weight are not unexpectedly dating models; Women are not able to have smaller dress sizes all of a sudden. Despite this dramatic increase in weight loss, there is no immediate acceptance into social circles. It causes a feeling of disappointment.

4. "Medicines and supplements can enhance your weight loss!"

Some people use medicines and miracle supplements to avoid starvation but eat less. Patients and friends ask me to give them phentermine at least 50 times a month. No one I know has used phentermine has experienced a significant weight loss, has not lost huge weight quantities, and the risk for treatment is great for people with an enlarged heart or elevated blood pressure. You should not take this with high blood pressure, atherosclerosis, glaucoma, or any heart condition already experienced by many obese people. The drug can cause restlessness, nervousness, dry mouth, and insomnia. However, people are so desperate to lose weight that they are still searching for artificial means of losing weight.

Worse still, in the last few years, I've had a few patients come to me to find that their use of fenfluramine medicine has, in the past, led to heart valve problems and lifelong heart disease. If you want to carry on believing that drugs and supplements are wonders of weight loss, you should prepare to give up huge amounts of money for minimal weight loss. Some supplements and medicines improve your weight loss, such as orlistat and phentermine. But to keep the results, you need to make sustainable changes. The findings are consistent and continuing with the methods I use and are methods of real life that the patient can understand without point calculations and higher mathematics, and no other person needs to buy the food processed and packed. You can use any food you want.

3. "French diets are tiny! This restaurant is gypping me!"

Let's now look at the quantities of food and how people joke about the little food French serve in their restaurants. Looking at pictures of people from the United States before 1960, you will see that we were then a lean country. People's dishes were smaller, we ate less food, and most of us were cut off. Look at the pictures of your mothers and your grandchildren — a photo worth 1000 words. People ate slightly and survived with thinner weight. Compare a plate from the restaurant to one now that you can get buffets from Atlantic City or Las Vegas. These are Big covers.

For these super-sized days, buffets, and large dinner plates, the mindset is quite different. These days we are expecting a full plate and expect second aid from what we need. We prefer succulent beverages. So the population as a whole wasn't as far removed from what we do in preparation, so exercise. Certainly, we have established extremely cross-training and extreme burning and core body preparation, but are it not funny how not all of these new regimes are different from past years. The only difference is that our conceptual desires have shifted to justify our grandparents' lean bodies to ourselves. Do you see in the museums fat skeletons of men and women?

France didn't go too far from previous eating habits. In reality, we constantly enjoy the small sizes of the French diet in American movies and advertisements. How they eat in part, however, is actually what is required. Only Google's "world obesity rankings," and you'll see where the United States and France stand now. You will see the USA at 30% obesity (3 out of 10 Americans obese), compared to France at 23, with 9.4% obesity (less than 1 out of 10). Mexico is 24 percent the nearest nation to the USA, and we're WAY above the rest of the world in the USA.

And now, the majority of the people are skeptical of the right amount of food on our diet. We have a food supply full of carbohydrates and high fructose corn syrup. Furthermore, we offer huge amounts of food for celebrations. The last wedding I was for 200 guests was five large tables of free alcohol and all-you-can-eat food. Move through the handful of food that we will eat. Christmas is still a gutbuster, and chocolate food is Easter and Halloween. Gluttony is now in vogue. Constant diet and drinking advertisements pounded the U.S. to create a regular amount of mega big burger, large fried, and large candy soda. We used to feed before we were exhausted instead of feeding when we were happy. Handfuls of food are natural and not excessive in the French diet! We don't have to be brainwashed until we're complete. We haven't heard our bodies stop eating when we're full. (This is one of the commands I send my clients to help lose weight). If you're hungry, stop if you're satisfied. Do not be full because that is the body's warning that you have gone too far.

Each of the above theories hinders proper weight management and rapid weight loss. They 're just a couple of the misconceptions that make people say nay when the doers lose weight with me. They think about "Frames" in Nitrolingual programming and hypnosis: these reference points people use for understanding the universe. The basic frame is optimistic versus pessimistic — do you think the glass is half empty or half full? Those who see the glass half full see the most things about their lives as optimistic, those who see it as half empty are cynical about what happens about their lives. Such views have been clouded over the years by physicians and patients on the right and wrong weight loss. When we reframe these ideas from commonly accepted truths to myths and obstacles to our success in weight loss, we accept that one pound is safe to lose each day by using our natural food intake reduction mechanism.

WEIGHT LOSS AND WOMEN: FAQ'S

What is the safest way to lose weight for women? But recent research has shown that women can lose weight differently than men.

What is the best way for me to lose weight?

Most women will need fewer calories to eat and drink and get the right amount of healthy food to lose weight. -- exercise or physical activity can help with weight loss, but others need to choose healthier foods (lean protein, whole grains, vegetables, and fruit). It is best to combine healthy food with increased physical activity. Speak to your doctor or health care professional before you begin a weight loss program. He or she can work with you to find the best way to lose weight for you.
Your environment and other areas of your life can make the loss of weight harder. You may be able to take other steps, such as talking to your doctor about any medications that might cause you weight gain, sleep gain, or stress, which may also help you lose weight.

How many calories should I eat and drink to lose weight safely?

Everyone is special. Everything is special. How fast you consume calories when you are not physically active can be very different from others depending on your particular genes, genetics, and personal experience. Whilst scientists are aware that 3,500 calories per pound exist, it's not always that you eat

500 fewer calories every day for a week (or 3,500 fewer calories a week).

Calories will help you lose weight if you have overweight or obese. Weight loss also happens when you concentrate on nutritious foods. Calories are usually derived from lean protein, whole grains, and fruits and vegetables and can safely reduce your weight.

There should be no diet of fewer than 800 calories a day for an adult woman. When you want to limit the number of calories, chat first to the doctor or nurse every day to lose weight. Your physician or nurse will help you find a safe and balanced number of calories for your body when attempting to lose weight. The precise amount of calories to aim depends on your age, height and weight, and how active you are.

Do women lose weight differently than men?

Yes and no. Yes and no. Often men lose weight faster than women. Yet weight loss typically varies between women and men over time.

People can lose weight faster as males generally have more muscle, and females can have more fat. Since muscle calories are consumed more than fat, men can burn more calories than women at rest.

Since men are on average heavier than women and have more supporting muscles, men typically eat more calories while still losing weight compared to women. For women, portion control may be particularly important. For one study, women who consumed less food (and fewer foods for general) had fewer BMIs than women who limited a certain food type or avoided it. This approach seems better for women than for men.

How does the menstrual cycle affect weight loss?

It does not appear that the menstrual cycle itself influences weight gain or loss. However, a period could influence your weight in other ways. Many people are suffering from premenstrual (PMS) syndrome. You can eat more sweet or salty foods than normal with PMS. These additional calories will lead to an increase in weight. And salt keeps the body to more water, which increases body weight (but not fat).

Although your menstrual cycle does not change the weight gain or loss, your menstrual cycle may be affected by losing or gaining weight. Women losing too much weight or losing weight too quickly can stop a period or have irregular periods. There may also be irregular periods for women with obesity. A daily duration is a sign of good health. A healthy weight can help women with irregular cycles to achieve more regular cycles.

How does menopause affect weight loss?

After menopause, it can be difficult to lose weight. Many women currently earn an average of 5 pounds after menopause. After menopause, lower estrogen levels can play a role in weight gain. Yet weight gains can be caused by a slowing down of the metabolism, less balanced eating habits, and less active age. When you grow old, you often lose muscle mass, and you consume fewer calories.

Staying active and eating healthy foods can help you keep track of your loss of weight.

How can I avoid gaining weight as I get older?

Women typically need fewer calories than men, particularly when they are old. It is because women have less muscle, more body fat, and typically are smaller than men. Adult women, on average, need between 1,600 and 2,400 calories a day. When you age, you have to take fewer calories to keep your weight even. You will also maintain your weight safely by increasing your physical activity.

Figure out how many calories your age and activity needs. You should also explore ways to eat better and get enough physical exercise with your doctor or nurse.

Can medications for weight loss help me lose weight?

Perhaps: Your doctor or nurse may recommend medicine for weight loss if:

- You have obesity (BMI of 30 or more)

OR

- You have overweight (27 or older BMI) and have additional weight-related health problems such as:

  o High blood pressure

  o High blood cholesterol

  o Diabetes

AND

- You count calories and do a lot of physical activity for at least six months but, on average, lose less than one pound a week.

The Food and Drug Administration has approved multiple medicines for obesity treatment. Many women who may get pregnant are not recommended because medicines can cause serious congenital disabilities in a baby.

Can over-the-counter or herbal weight-loss drugs help me lose weight?

Perhaps, nine but always talk to your physician or nurse before you take any herbal or dietary supplements. Find your main ingredient on this fact sheet in your supplement to see if it works and is safe.

There is no guarantee that weight loss products "herbal" or "natural" are safe for everyone. The administration of food and drugs does not regulate additives in the same way as it regulates medicines. Additives often have side effects and can interfere with your medicine.

What surgical options are used to treat obesity?

Operations for weight loss – also known as bariatric operations – can help treat obesity. A doctor can recommend weight-loss surgical treatment if you:

- • Have a 40 or higher Body Mass Index (BMI)

- • have 35 or greater BMI and health conditions linked to weight, such as heart disease or diabetes

Bariatric operation is not a "quick fix," but a major operation.

Is liposuction treatment for obesity?

Liposuction is not an obesity treatment. Fat is removed from under the skin during this operation. Liposuction may be used to reshape body parts. But if you gain weight after the operation, fat will go back to the places where you have had an operation or grow elsewhere.

I carry extra weight, but I'm fit. Do I still need to lose weight?

You are lucky to be healthy and take steps to improve your health! Sometimes your body mass index (BMI) can indicate that, although you are fit, you are overweight. And some people can argue that it is more important how physically active you are than how much extra weight you bear.
This is only partially true, however. Being physically active can reduce your risk of heart disease, even without losing weight.10 Your risk may be higher than that of someone exercising and having a healthy weight. In other words, being healthy does not reduce the dangers of overweight.
Speak to your doctor or nurse about your healthy weight.

How fast should I try to lose weight?

It can be tempting to follow a "crash" diet and quickly lose loads of pounds. But women who slowly lose weight are more likely to keep it hidden. Discuss your priorities with your doctor or nurse. Your doctor or nurse can assist you in developing a healthy diet and activity plan.

I've lost weight but have hit a plateau. How do I continue losing weight?

After losing weight at a rate of up to 1 pound a week for about six months, most people hit a plateau or weight that does not fall anymore. When you lose weight, your restful metabolism (how many calories you burn) falls. Your body needs fewer calories to sustain itself at a lower weight.

After about six months, many people will lose about 10% of their original body weight. If you want to continue losing weight, the number of calories you eat and drink each day, and your physical activity may need to be adjusted.

If you eat healthy foods but still experience weight, you may want to talk to a physician who is specialized in obesity or weight management (the link is external). It can also be difficult to hold away the weight you have gained.

CONCLUSION

Every other day, new weight loss techniques are invented. Earlier, it was when workouts were all decorated with leotards and spandex costumes when making music, then came to the age of yoga, which was quite soon overtaken by power yoga. After this, muscle building was seen as the only way to deal with weight loss. There were countless methods such as these, but the new method of weight reduction by hypnosis is an entirely different experience.

Those who think hypnosis does not require physical labor but loses weight of the mind will be disappointed. Hypnosis helps to lose weight by keeping the mind and bodyweight-loss targets. Nearly all ages and sexes, whether male or female, young or old, have been reported as having trouble controlling weight. There are concerns about increasing obesity problems. The issue is no longer limited to the Hollywood idea of body size or weight loss.

However, this issue is that doctors want their patients to lose weight because heart disease, diabetes, and many other types of problems are rising. But it would appear that these people are not guilty of eating all kinds of fast food and that they are satisfied in their current situation. Doctors don't want their patients to stop eating junk food but want to reduce their consumption of health benefits. However, most people are not sufficiently motivated to lose weight.

Obesity causes women to become fascinated with yo-yo diets and fading diets. Such diets include the cycle of taking a diet, losing a couple of pounds, but not going on and getting off the diet. As a result, the lost pounds return easier. Again, the dieter starts a new diet, and the cycle goes on and becomes an endless chain. This repeated weight loss and increase will lead to a rough ride in the metabolism of the body. This often profoundly influences the dietitian.

A new approach has been created for this health issue. This

involves hypnosis, which motivates the body and mind to concentrate on weight loss. As a result, the body attempts to avoid unhealthy foods and yo-yo diets but continues to focus on losing weight healthily. The psychologist or therapist maintains the patient motivated by the constant Hypnose method towards the health loss program.

The key purpose of hypnosis is to enter the unconscious mind and attempt to control the conscious level of thought. In the meantime, the unconscious handles the automatic items that involve binding the shoes and other associated tasks. The subconscious is the driving power that works on the conscious brain to control our actions and, thus, weight loss without fading diets.

CPSIA information can be obtained
at www.ICGtesting.com
Printed in the USA
BVHW081531070521
606759BV00010B/1766